So, What Are You Calling It?
The joys and perils of naming your child
Alex Lee and Brendan Moffett

CYANBOOKS

For Mam, Darcy, Callum, Holly, Vaughn, Tara and Finn

Copyright © 2005 Swell Ideas Ltd

First published in Great Britain in 2005 by
Cyan Books, an imprint of

Cyan Communications Limited
119 Wardour Street
London
W1F 0UW
T: +44 (0)20 7565 6120
E: sales@cyanbooks.com
www.cyanbooks.com

The right of Alex Lee and Brendan Moffett
to be identified as the authors of this work
has been asserted by them in accordance
with the Copyright, Designs and Patents
Act 1988.

All rights reserved

No part of this publication may be
reproduced, stored in a retrieval system
or transmitted in any form or by any
means including photocopying, electronic,
mechanical, recording or otherwise,
without the prior written permission of the
rights holders, application for which must
be made to the publisher.

A CIP record for this book is available from
the British Library

ISBN 1-904879-39-X

Designed by R&D&Co
Printed and bound in Great Britain by
TJ International, Padstow, Cornwall

Contents

Chapter 1: page 5
No going back: How naming your child affects its life
Chapter 2: page 19
Don't be a Dick: The perils of nicknaming
Chapter 3: page 31
Tribal gathering
Chapter 4: page 43
Born famous: How to give your child star quality
Chapter 5: page 57
Scrabbling around: If you're not religious, why not make up a name?
Chapter 6: page 85
Team player: If the name fits, wear it on your football shirt
Chapter 7: page 97
My future's so bright, I gotta wear shades: The phuture of naming
Chapter 8: page 117
The great divide: Names that don't travel
Chapter 9: page 133
Kojak and other Telly names
Chapter 10: page 151
Silly-brity kids' names
Chapter 11: page 165
Chardonnay, madam? The world of the chav

No going back: How naming your child affects its life

1

What do you call a man with a truck on his head?

Laurie!

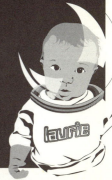

As a parent, your list of responsibilities to your newborn child is an immensely long and arduous, some would say torturous, one. Aside from the obvious stuff –

DON'T LET IT SHOVE DANGEROUS OBJECTS IN ITS MOUTH OR LEAVE IT IN A SITUATION WHERE IT MIGHT SUFFOCATE (THERE'S NOTHING YOU CAN DO ABOUT THIS IF IT GROWS UP TO BE AN MP)

FEED, WASH AND CLEAN IT REGULARLY

KEEP IT WARM

WATCH IT DOESN'T FALL ON ITS HEAD TOO OFTEN

SHOW IT OFF TO FRIENDS AND RELATIVES AS IF IT WERE THE FIRST BABY EVER TO HAVE BEEN BORN

TALK COMPLETE NONSENSE TO IT FOR AT LEAST THE FIRST TWO YEARS OF ITS LIFE

– and so on, you need to give it a name that'll ease its passage through life: its first day at school, its first day at work or college, the moment it meets the person it falls in love with, the time when it has to sign its first cheque, the first time it gets points on its driving licence and all those other pivotal life events.

This book is an invaluable aid to making the right decision

about naming your child. Let's face it, there have been plenty of times in your life when you've hated your parents for no other reason than giving you a daft, too long, too short, irrelevant, unsuitable, silly, ridiculous, embarrassing, ordinary, crazy, humbling, meaningless, worthless (delete as appropriate) name. *So, What Are You Calling It?* will guide you safely and decisively towards giving your child the moniker it'll be saddled with until it is old enough to understand the term "deed poll." Within these pages, you'll be advised on the complete process to follow in order to name your child successfully, thus leaving no opportunity for ridicule, confusion or embarrassment in the years to come.

Please don't underestimate the importance of reading this book from beginning to end. You wouldn't read the Bible and miss out Revelations, thumb through *Pride and Prejudice* without relishing the bit where Mr Darcy snogs Elizabeth Bennett for the first time, or skip the page in *Oliver Twist* where the young scamp asks the master for more. Leave a chapter or even a page unturned and your child may get the wrong name. Nigel, say. What sort of name is that to call a girl?

OK, let's start with the fundamentals: some ground rules that will stand you in good stead once you know for definite the type of nappies you're going to have to buy the kid and what colour you need to repaint its bedroom.

The first rule of naming a child is *Keep it simple*. And the second, and the third. (If a fourth rule were to exist, it'd be too complicated.) Face it, the kid's lumbered with the name you give it for the rest of its life. It didn't ask to be born, but if it could speak from the safety of the womb it would say, "OK, so I'm going to be born, I can accept that, but please don't saddle me with a ridiculous name that's going to ruin my life." How do you think it's going to cope if it can't even pronounce or spell its own name?

So folks, keep it simple. There is of course a formula to this minimalist approach. The fewer letters the better; the fewer syllables the better (three at the most); and the quicker you can say it, the better. You're allowed a maximum of nine letters (ten's just plain greedy) and a minimum of three, which gives rise to the following formula:

N = >2 <10L x <4S

where N = name, L = number of letters and S = number of syllables.

Any other formula is, quite simply, a formula for disaster.

Any would-be child namer can use this formula to stay within the bounds of reasonable child-naming behaviour. In fact, this formula should be indelibly etched into every birth certificate. That way, the registrar can make an informed decision as to whether to agree to commit any given name onto a document that could easily make or break the child's life.

Picture the scene. Man, woman and screaming child enter registrar's office to register the birth of their child.

"What a lovely looking little girl," remarks the registrar, desperately trying to sound sincere as the baby vomits, lets out blood-curdling screams and wets herself on a rota strictly determined by the number of times she hears the words "Ssshh" and "There's a good girl." "And what will you be naming her today?"

"Emilinniah," reply the doting parents in stereo.

"Sorry, folks, but I ain't writing that on the birth certificate. You'll have to try again," says the registrar, safe in the knowledge that she has the power of the formula to back her up.

"Why not? It's our choice," says the disbelieving mother, handing the baby to the gob-smacked father.

"Yup, but you've contravened the formula. Too many letters, too many syllables. Sorry. Next!"

On the other hand, other formulas for naming your child haven't quite stood the time. Take for example

$E = MC^2$

which of course means

Egbert = Moniker Chosen is Stupid

and

$dx / \{a^2 - x^2\} = \arcsin(x/a) + \text{const.}$

and

$dx/\{a2 + x2\} = (1/a)$ arctan (x/a) + const.

which roughly translates as "If you want your child to stand any chance of becoming a mathematical genius, don't waste your time thinking of a name for it; let it work out one for itself, and as soon as it can spell its own name, get it to sign over a percentage of its future earnings to you."

Staying on the theme of simplicity, please, whatever you do, don't mess about with the order of your children's names. It'll mentally scar them for life, and they'll end up hating you for it. The reason why first names are called first names is because they're first. It stands to reason, then, that middle names go in the middle and last names take their rightful place at the end of the queue.

Messing about with the order of your child's name will cause untold grief from the moment your child and its friends learn how to speak, and will haunt your child long into adulthood and no doubt create annoying, unnecessary and ultimately deeply upsetting administrative complications at its funeral.

Take, for example, the name of the author of this book: James Alexander Lee. A boring, ordinary name, yes? Well, yes, but his name is Alex." Why Alex?" people ask him. Does he not like James or something? What's wrong with James? It was good enough for several kings of England.

Stop it! Let the man explain.

His father and grandfather were both called James, and his mother and father wanted to carry on the tradition. Nothing wrong with that, but they also wanted to call their son Alexander. Fair dos. Nothing wrong with that either. So why not first name James, middle name Alexander? Simple! Oh no. Nothing so straightforward, obvious or just plain sensible for Mr and Mrs Lee. Call him James Alexander, but *use his middle name as his first name*.

So young James Alexander toddles off for his first day at school, teetering under the weight of his backpack, half choking to death by elastic tie and unsure whether to bend his arms for fear of ruining his brand-new school shirt.

He goes into the classroom to join thirty other scared young children. But he's different from them all. He knows it. They don't know it yet, but boy, will they find out soon enough.

Immediately, confusion reigns.

"What's your first name?" asks the teacher, a well-meaning middle-aged lady who loves kids, wears glasses and does everything by the book.

"Errr..." wonders our Alex. Does the little lad go for Alexander when he knows full well that he would be lying if he said Alexander and that lying's really bad and he won't go to heaven, and . . . and . . . and . . . Or does he go for James knowing that one day he's going to have to correct his teacher in front of the whole class and admit his real name to everyone, thus heaping embarrassment upon himself and opening himself up to ridicule for the rest of his days from his friends *whose names are in the proper order*?

"Come on, don't be shy, everyone has to say their name in front of the class. It's a way of getting to know each other better," coaxes the teacher.

Now the whole class – and quite possibly the whole school – is staring at James Alexander, and he doesn't like it.

He flicks an imaginary coin in his head. Heads I'll say Alexander; tails and it's James. Flick! The coin flies up in the air and starts spinning. Heads, tails, heads, tails, heads, tails, faster and faster until it bounces on the floor. Three times. It's heads. Whatever happened to "Tails never fails?" Alexander is such a difficult word to say for a four-year-old boy. Come on, deep breath...

"Alexander," he finally replies in his best, clearest, least nervous, most manly voice.

The teacher, momentarily distracted by the young male student teacher walking past the window, regains her concentration.

"Alexandra?"

The classroom erupts. More than one child actually wets itself laughing. Ha ha! No wonder he wouldn't say his name! He's got a girl's name! Ha ha ha! Girl's name! Girl's name!

"No," he replies, in the most forceful tone a quivering four-year-old nervous wreck can muster, "it's Alexan-DERR."

To be fair to the teacher, she doesn't make an issue of this.

"And have you got a middle name, Alexander?"

Oh, for God's sake...

OK, so you've had a bit of a think as to how to name your child. You're going to keep it simple: if you are going to give it a middle name, it'll be in the middle. Your child will be known by its first name. You've achieved two of the fundamentals already, but there's a long, long way to go before making its name official. So stop and think for a moment.

Ask yourself these questions:

We both like this name, but *why* do we both like it? Do we really both like it or is one of us just keeping quiet for the sake of an easy life? Where have we heard this name before? Who else has it?

Now you're beginning to sniff what you should be smelling. Everyone's had to contend with the "Ha ha, oh yeah, such and such blah" moment. It sends a shiver down your spine, the "Ha ha, oh yeah, such and such blah" moment. We've all experienced it at least once in our lives. If you're asked to recall the time, date and what you were wearing on that uncomfortable, nerve-jarring occasion, you'll know right away. It's a feeling you'll never quite shake off for the rest of your life.

Picture the scene. You and your partner proudly introduce your child to someone for the first time.

"So what are you calling it?" (good title for a book, yes?) asks the interested party.

"Michael," you reply, knowing what's coming next...

"Ha ha, oh yeah, Michael Jackson!"

or **"Ha ha, oh yeah, Michael Crawford!"**

or **"Ha ha, oh yeah, Michael Winner!"**

or **"Ha ha, oh yeah, Michael Owen!"**

The dreaded "Ha ha, oh yeah, such and such blah" moment. Avoid it at all costs. It's your solemn duty. Now you're thinking, oh my God, is there nothing I can name my child that will see it safely through the rigours of life?

Well, relax and put your feet up. In fact, make a cup of tea first. There are plenty of names you can safely name your child so it won't grow up hating you. The "Ha ha, oh yeah, such and such blah" moment will seem like a short walk in a particularly pleasant park compared to the stress you and your child will have to endure if you name it incorrectly. But, you ask, how do I know if it's correct or not?

Easy. Give the child a head start by spelling its name properly. Why do some parents insist on spelling their child's name wrong? Time to be blunt: they're illiterate, have no class or didn't want to have the screaming little shitbag. There are no excuses. Stephen is spelt that way for a reason: because it's the right spelling. Ditto Steven. There are two ways to spell Stephen/Steven, but only two. Don't ever forget that. If you decide your child is to be named Steeven, Steephen, Stieven, Stephyn, Stevyn or any other frankly preposterous variation on the proper spellings, shame on you. It's you who deserve the stick, the name-calling and the humiliation, not your child. If you're ever in any doubt about how to spell your child's name, *don't name it that way* – it's stupid and the joke's on you. Although, to be fair, your child will get all the aggro, and hey, it's not as if you wanted it in the first place.

But seriously, folks, picking a child's name is of the utmost importance. How would you like it if you had a rubbish name? Many of you reading this *will* have a rubbish name, whether you care to admit it or not, and you'll want to avoid what your parents did to you when you were born, that is saddle your child with a name so embarrassing that you'd rather be known as Squiggle. Next time you see someone sign their name, take a look: nine times out of ten that's exactly what it'll say. Because their parents gave them a nauseating name. Which brings us nicely to another vitally important rule to bear in mind when naming your child:

Don't use alliteration. It's only clever when used by poets. A later chapter will cover the folly of a famous footballing father and the idiocy of an Icelandic quizmaster's parents. Where naming your child is concerned, alliteration is the territory of the terrible, the arena of the awful and the region of the ridiculous. If your surname is Smith, don't call your child Sammy. The fact it's a brand of beer's a good enough reason, never mind what images the initials SS might conjure up for people old enough to remember the war.

Names should be memorable for their simplicity, not because they reflect the qualities of your surname in some way. Who wants to be remembered as a full name anyway? And there's another factor to work into your naming equation: stop and think how the people around your child may alter its name. A non-alliterative first name could suddenly be dragged into the mire of alliteration by ancient nicknaming convention. Never lose sight of the fact that William can become Bill, Robert can be altered to Bobby and Richard can always be changed to Dick. Mr and Mrs Head pay particular attention; sometimes alliteration is the least of your worries. Remember – a name is for life, not just for Christmas.

Before you rush off to the next chapter or, worse, to the local register office to commit your child to a life of comedy-name-induced woe, consider this. When you mention your child's name in conversation, does the person you're talking to realize you're talking about your child, or do they think you're talking about one of your pets?

It's happened before, it's happening now and it'll happen again. It's inexcusable. Dogs, cats, goldfish and so forth are allowed stupid names. In fact, they *deserve* stupid names and it's your duty to give them stupid names. However macho Butch, Spike or Bruno might sound, they're dogs' names. In fact, they're *cartoon* dogs' names. How would you like to share your name with that of a dumb animated pooch that's destined to be thwarted by a stealthier mouse or a more cunning cat for ever and a day? There's nothing big or clever about it. So what if your baby boy looked a bit on the tough side when he was born, or you wanted to exorcize yourself vicariously of your own less than macho moniker?

Giving your boy a girl's name will make his life even tougher. Just ask Marion Morrison or Shirley Crabtree – via a safe, organized séance run by a professional medium. They'll be happy to tell you all about their tough-guy lives.

Sources
http://www.fidnet.com/~dap1955/dickens/twist_more.html
http://www.dreambeliever.org/impressions.html

Don't be a Dick: The perils of nicknaming

2

What do you call someone who hangs around in bushes?

Russell!

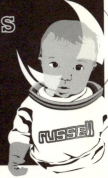

"OK, so what are you calling it?" asks your best mate (and they haven't even read the book yet). You nervously reply, "Oh I don't know yet, I'll leave it to the wife/husband/vicar to decide" when secretly you know exactly what your child is going to be called and it's so bad you're too embarrassed to say. Well there's still hope, because for every abysmal name there's a great nickname.

You'll know this already, but a nickname is a short, clever, mundane, obvious, cute, derogatory or otherwise substitute name for a person or thing's real name (for example, Nick is short for Nicholas). It is therefore different from a pseudonym, which is generally used in order to mask one's identity, though there can of course be an overlap between the two. (This occurs only in extreme cases when someone hates their name so much that their pseudonym becomes their nickname or, conversely, when someone's nickname is so far removed from their real name that it becomes their pseudonym. Whatever.) Let's have a look at some nicknames because even if you act with the best intentions of bestowing upon your child a good, solid, noble-sounding, correctly spelt name, its nickname may give you nightmares.

By the way, if you really want to show off, here's how the word nickname originated. And no, it's not because long, long ago everyone was called Nicholas. That would just be stupid (although having said that, it was good enough for about 600 consecutive tsars of Russia).

In Middle English, the term used for nickname was *ekename*. This, perversely, came from eke, meaning addition. Which is a bit daft, as surely the purpose of a nickname is to save valuable nanoseconds of breath, not add extra ones? Well, not always; just spend a few seconds flicking through your brain to come up with a few nicknames your friends and family have had to endure over the years. By the way, in Swedish, the word *öknamn* translates literally as nickname. (Admittedly that's only of any use whatsoever if you go to pub quizzes. In Stockholm.) Anyway, the word *ekename* developed into nickname. Why? Simple. People couldn't resist giving *ekename* a nickname. Nickname's easier to say, you see. Try saying it, you know this much is true: it saves a good three nanoseconds of valuable talking time.

In Viking societies, many people had nicknames such as Heiti, Viðrnefni or Uppnefi which were used as well as, or instead of, their family names. In some circumstances, the giving of a nickname had a special status in Viking society. It created a relationship between the nicknamer and the nicknamee, to the extent that it often entailed a formal ceremony and an exchange of gifts. (In fact, very much like a modern-day wedding, except without the ridiculously expensive wedding list, embarrassing best man's speech and rows over the seating arrangements.)

You wouldn't believe how many different types of nickname there are. Let's start with the easiest one: the first-name nickname, which is of vital importance to you as a potential child namer. You'll soon understand why.

Even first-name nicknames can come in all shapes and sizes. The easiest way to use them is simply to shorten your child's name. So, as a general rule of thumb, don't call them anything daft like William, Penistone or Cheesybellendi. Yeah, OK, the last one's made up. And the second is a village in Derbyshire.

Right then, erm . . . a first-name nickname relates directly, as you'd rightly expect, to a person's first name. There are many obvious examples, but it's better to be safe than sorry and not assume anything about the parent (i.e. you) that is about to name their child. To make your choice idiot-proof, here are some samples of first names along with nicknames and surnames that you might have not realized would combine in a less than funny way with your new child's nickname:

Ali (Allison): Baba, Minyum, Bye
Andy (Andrew): and Pandy
Bill (William): Abong
Bob (Robert): Ajob
Charlie (Charles): Snorter
Donna (Donnatella): Kebab
Ted (Edward): Ebear
Jack (John): Spratt, Frost,
  Benimblejackbequickjackjumpoverthecandlestick
Nat (Nathan): Ralbornkiller
Nell (Eleanor): Eethelephant
Peggy, Maggie, Meg, Marge (Margaret):
  Sue, Mae, Abyte, Simpson
Ron (Ronald): Dayvoo
Sam (Samantha): Harriton
Steve (Stephen): Anidge
Sue (Susan): Baroo

Admittedly some of the surnames are slightly on the outlandish side, but you get the idea. Name your child with a name that can be shortened at your peril. You never know what it might lead to.

Nicknames come from surnames as well as first names, of course. You'll think yourself lucky, as will your child when it grows up, if you've got a decent nicknamable surname. Let's look at a few.

Someone with the surname Mitchell can end up being called *Mitch*, just as a Sullivan can be known as *Sully*. There are countless examples, many of which actually *extend* the person's surname, thus adding effort on the nicknamer's behalf but also slightly dehumanizing the nicknamee by ignoring the fact that they have a first name. You know, like when a teacher, sergeant-major or boss insists on calling you by an extra-syllabic comedy version of your surname: Binns becomes Binno, Hazeltine Hazelteenee, Lee Lee-o. All good harmless fun, but worth noting nonetheless.

By now you should have realized that your responsibility as a child namer extends beyond the simple premise of "Ooh, that's a nice name, that'll do." Never assume anything when you name your child; in particular, don't overlook the effortless creativity that cruel peers will deploy to render your child's first name irrelevant. But how? you ask. Easy: they make up a surname-based nickname for your child that it won't shake off for the rest of its life.

There's basically nothing you can do about this particular sort of nickname, so just live with it and concentrate on not giving your child a less than perfect first name. Having said that, there's no harm in pointing out a few instances of what might happen to your child's surname when manipulated by the minds of minors. Just to prepare you for the worst, you understand.

If your child's surname is White, for example, its nickname could be any of the following: Chalky, Blackie, Whitey, Eggy or Shitey. Harsh maybe, but your eyes need opening to the facts. Brace yourself for some more surname nicknames. A child with the surname Bird might as well forget about ever being called by its real first name outside the four walls of its parental home. It will be saddled with the name Dicky, Lass, Woman, Big, Tweety Pie or something equally preposterous. Which in many ways is worse than having a rubbish name.

To be perfectly clear on this vitally important issue: *never lose sight of your child's surname* as it can be twisted into something so rank and rancid (but nonetheless consistently hilarious in the playground/workplace) that the name you decide on for your kid will become meaningless and irrelevant. There's only one way out of this nightmare scenario: give your child a first name that starts or ends with the letter V, X or Z and has a Y somewhere in the middle. Treat yourself to a big pat on the back if it's totally unpronounceable, even by visiting aliens.

That's not to say that the possibility of your child copping for the nickname from hell (Beelzebub, anyone?) ends there. Once it grows up and gets a job, its line of work can determine what nickname it receives.

Chip is a regular nickname for carpenters, particularly if they've got a penchant for French fries and enjoy the fineries of golf. On the other hand, if your child ever rises to a position of power or authority, it can reasonably expect to acquire a number of nicknames, with the redeeming factor that it may never get to hear any of them said to its face. Even travel is not without its risks. If your child ever moves to another part of the country or indeed the world it will encounter a whole bunch of nicknames – often offensive, or simply just demeaning – based purely on where people come from.

Everyone has heard Oz for an Australian, or indeed Ozzie for a shaky-handed heavy-metal star with a dysfunctional family. People hailing from New Zealand are branded Kiwis, whereas Brits are known as Limeys if they're in the US or Poms if they're in Australia. When it comes to international travel, no one's bothered about your first name, only where you're from. This is one of the few occasions where your choice of your child's name is completely irrelevant, so if you've got an inexplicable urge to call your child something a little ker-azy, you're allowed to as long as you make those emigration plans quickly.

If you're not planning on leaving the country quite yet, you need to heed the following advice too: *don't give your child a name that readily pairs up with an undesirable physical characteristic*. This needs explanation. Giving your child a decent name is one of the best things you can do for it. One of the other things you can do that your offspring will thank you for in later life is to give it a balanced diet. In other words, don't let it get too fat or too skinny, as the name you've pigeon-holed it with may pair up with its undesirable physical attribute in the same way that tea (six sugars, naturally) pairs up with scones (of the low-fat variety, to counterbalance the sugar).

Here are a few examples of nicknames that fat people may face at some point in their cake-guzzling lives: Tubby, Fatso, Lardarse, Chubby. So if you name your child Terry, Freddie, Larry or Charlotte they could end up with an alliterative nightmare of a nickname. Conversely, if you're one of those parents who'd sooner force-feed their child carrot sticks than give in and take them to the nearest drive-in McBurger outlet, your kid could end up with the sobriquet Skinny, Matchstick, Bones, Cambodian or worse. So out goes Samantha, Michael, Barbara, Callum and any other names beginning with those letters. Be careful – it's a jungle out there. Bear in mind our guidelines, be aware how onerous a task naming a child is, and above all, don't let it get fat or thin at any point in its life. It just isn't worth it.

Another fascinating nicknaming convention that illustrates how clever we all are is the opposite nickname. We've heard them all before, but it's our duty to warn you about all the pitfalls, so here's a quick reminder:

**SLIM FOR FATTIES
SHORTY FOR GIANTS
LOFTY FOR TITCHES
BLUE FOR GINGER-HAIRED FOLK
AND SO ON.**

Woe betide you if your child ever develops a noticeable personality trait and a nicknamer picks up on it. Once again, your child's first name will go straight out the window. The merest hint of a temper will earn it the nickname Grumpy, the first signs of academic achievement will induce a Swotty, and if you have a young lad who becomes a bit of a ladies' man (admit it, fellas, you all secretly want this for your sons), then he'll become Romeo faster than you can say "Hey Tarquin, get off that phone."

Finally, and most important, whatever name you give your child, don't expect it to last for ever. You now know nearly all (yup, *nearly* all) the traps you could fall into when it comes to nicknaming. By all means bear them in mind when you're making your naming decision, but be realistic. Resign yourself to the fact that your child will do something at some point in its life that someone will notice, and that something will be sufficiently funny, controversial or downright daft that its first name will henceforth become an irrelevance.

Even the author of this book, who has led a sheltered, almost hermit-like existence, is acquainted with a number of people who are known only by nicknames that they've picked up through doing something that somebody else couldn't resist commemorating. Take Des (real name

Andrew), who once mispronounced something in French; Jim-jams (real name John), who wore paisley pyjamas on a school trip; and Butty (real name David), who once nutted someone on a building site.

To sum up, come to an agreement about your child's name, name it thus, and don't ever let it out of the house afterwards. There's a nicknamer lurking on every corner.

Sources
http://www.funnynames.com/
http://www.weirdnames.com/

Tribal gathering

3

Why has Edward Woodward got four Ds in his name?

'Cos if he didn't, he'd be called E-war Woo-war!

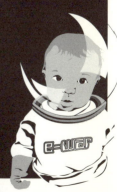

As the late lamented Elvis Aron (or Aaron, depending on which funeral stonemason you use) Presley once said about naming children, "Wise men say only fools rush in." OK, so the King wasn't really singing about naming kids, but his words offer the soundest of advice on this topic.

Naming conventions differ from country to country. We may be familiar with a certain set of rather staid, ritualistic conventions (admit it, you've followed them yourself, or fallen victim to them):

NAME HIM AFTER HIS FATHER
NAME HER AFTER HER GRANDMOTHER
NAME HIM AFTER THE CITY IN WHICH HE WAS CONCEIVED
NAME HER AFTER A FLOWER
NAME HIM AFTER A FIGURE FROM THE BIBLE
NAME HER AFTER OUR FAVOURITE POP STAR
... AND SO ON.

But these time-honoured practices aren't universal; millions of people worldwide have different ideas. Let's examine a few other methods from places and cultures you may otherwise never encounter. You never know, you might learn something.

Native Americans (don't call them Red Indians – they're not red, nor are they Indians) have the naming of children off to a T. Although a child is generally named within a few days of its birth, a person may have numerous names during its lifetime. Imagine that! No sooner do you get used to being known as Little Running Water when you suddenly become Big Chief Stomping Tree. Or something. Just to add that extra ingredient of confusion, the tradition and practice of naming an individual vary from tribe to tribe.

This is why it's fundamentally wrong to slag off other people behind their backs in native American society. For all you know, the tribespeople you were bad-mouthing earlier could have changed their names in the meantime, and loads of *other* tribespeople could have changed *their* names to the ones you were using during your back-biting session. Suddenly the insults you were hurling at little weedy Native Americans start applying to people who are much bigger and harder than they were, and own much sharper axes.

There's always a get-out clause, though. You can use the excuse *that* you didn't mean that Little Jumping Pony, you meant the *other* Little Jumping Pony. Native Americans don't have family names, so they needn't worry about such niceties as rhyming or alliterative surnames. Having said that, it's best not to get into a linguistic debate about Native American naming traditions when a strapping six-footer with a Mohican is heading your way doing a war dance and waving a big axe around his head.

In Native American society, names bestowed at birth by a grandparent are often taken from a respected predecessor. Later in life, names earned through deeds may be derived from a dream or a vision quest. For Plains Indians and people of other regions, the childhood name is changed in a special ceremony at the time of passage to adulthood, after which a dream name may be used.

The term Hanblecheyapi or Hanbleceya, which means *crying for a vision*, denotes the vision quest of the Sioux Indians. An oft-heard conversation in Sioux tribes goes as follows:

Mother: What are you crying for?
Son: I'm crying for a vision!
Mother: I'll vision you in a minute, now get in this wigwam and practise your smoke signals!

Native Americans look to visions to give them guidance in choosing a name. The vision quest ritual lasts for many days, and consists of isolation, fasting and exposure to the elements. Individuals usually strip naked, paint their bodies with clay, purify themselves in a sweat lodge and then retreat into isolation for a long fast. The vision can come in the form of an animal, an ancestor, a plant, an object, a location or an act of nature such as a storm – or a particularly loud fart. Those who have gone on a quest then relate their experiences to a shaman who can help to interpret the symbolism involved.

Parents send boys and girls out on vision quests from the age of four until puberty, in the same way that we send our children out for cigarettes. Although it's most common among the young, people may seek a spiritual vision at many times during their lives, even when they are old – a bit like going to the pub, really.

At twenty days old, infants from the Hopi people take part in a traditional ceremony where they are dedicated to the sun, then given their names. Perhaps this explains why so many native Indian children are called Sunny at some stage in their lives.

If you are lucky enough to be born into a wealthy man's family among the north-west coast Salish tribes, there will be a massive, boozy celebration to announce your name to the world. In Ireland, one family has a boy who now boasts 23 names. The father is looking forward to celebrating his son's first birthday.

Most Indians of the Plains tribes take on a new name only after they have committed an act to demonstrate their prowess, as in Great Brave Bear Slayer. All most Brits have to do is wait for their friends to stick a "y" on their surname.

The traditions in Surinam are somewhat different. Babies are named according to the time, circumstances and place of their birth. They are often given ancestral names in the belief that this brings long-dead forebears back to life. Children may also be named after heroes, parents or siblings. To safeguard newborn babies against inheriting the spirits of dubious individuals, children can't be named after a murderer, rapist or other criminal; nor can they be named after known wizards. You wouldn't find any Sutcliffes, Bundys or Merlins troubling Surinam registrars.

Traditions vary from tribe to tribe. Among members of the Bukusus, a son born to a mother who dies in childbirth is named *Kundu*, meaning monster (slightly harsh, but never mind), Makokha, or *rubbish* (hey, come on) or Nasimiyu, or *hyena* (well, you've got to laugh, haven't you?) The

Luos call a child who is born on the road Ayoo (girl) or Oyoo (boy). A child born at night is named Atieno/Otieno, in the morning Akinyi/Omondi, at noon Anyango/Onyango, and in the evening Odhiambo/Adhiambo. All very straightforward. But it's probably a good job that western culture doesn't observe this particular tradition. If someone round your way comes up with a ridiculous name for their kid, at least they had a bit of choice in the matter, and weren't stuck with calling it Day, Night or Lunchtime.

The practices that accompany naming include dressing the baby with charms to protect it from witchcraft and other evils (the rough equivalent of chav parents getting their kids' ears pierced when they're, like, six months old and forcing them to wear sovereign rings on their fingers from the age of one). Special food is given to the mother and the baby, presents are given to the baby as a sign of welcome and acceptance of the name, and sacrifices are performed to thank God and ask him for protection. Once again, these traditions aren't as far removed from ours as we might think. We give babies presents; for special food, read beer/wine/spirits; and as for sacrifices, well, in the UK fathers often vow to stay away from the pub more often.

Among the Luhya, newborn babies are given millet porridge. If they die, the powers that be conclude that they were not part of the community. Again a bit harsh, you might think, but hey, if a kid can't take its porridge it doesn't deserve to live, let alone be given a decent name. All the above may seem somewhat strange to people like us who take running water, fresh bread and Burberry for granted, but what you've just read pales into insignificance when compared to the way that Kenya's largest ethnic group, the Kikuyu, go about naming each other.

The Kikuyu tribe was originally founded by a man named Gikuyu (go figure where his parents plucked *that* name from). Kikuyu history says that the Kikuyu god, Ngai (so called because he was a guy), took Gikuyu to the top of Kirinyaga and told him to stay and build his home there. He was also given his wife, Mumbi (yes, even then women spoke mumbo-jumbo). Mumbi and Gikuyu had ten daughters, but as the Kikuyu considered it bad luck to say the number ten out loud, they never admitted it. When counting they used to say "full nine" instead of ten. It was from the nine daughters that the nine Kikuyu clans – Achera, Agachiku, Airimu, Ambui, Angare, Anjiru, Angui, Aithaga and Aitherandu – were formed.

In Kikuyu culture, family identity is perpetuated by naming the first boy after the father's father and the second after the mother's father. The same principle applies to the girls. The first is named after the father's mother and the second after the mother's mother. Try explaining that when you've had a few. Subsequent children are named after the grandparents' brothers and sisters, starting with the oldest and working down to the youngest. Members of the tribe believed that the spirit of a dead grandparent would inhabit the new child who took their name. (This belief was blown out of the water when life expectancy rose; these days grandparents are often still around when their grandchildren are born.)

Still in Kenya, the Kamba community follows a different set of traditions. Women in labour are assisted by a birth attendant called a Mwithakya (luckily, it's not a name you'd use regularly) who also helps choose the baby's name. This can be selected from two sources: a hereditary pool of the names of deceased family members and friends, or a circumstantial pool relating to the circumstances of the child's birth. Whether any Kamba names translate directly as Difficult, Induced, Messy or Ouch, That Bloody Hurt isn't known.

There are names for babies born prematurely, after their due date or on the way to the birth attendant's home. Other names refer to the weather or other aspects of nature: for example, Wambua is a name given to a boy born on a rainy day, and Symbua is the girl's equivalent. Thankfully this tradition isn't followed in Manchester, or else there'd be mass confusion in class whenever the teacher read out the register.

In *African Religions and Philosophy*, J. S. Mbiti explains that the Luo tribes choose a name for a newborn baby while it is crying. They call out the names of living or dead people, and if the baby stops crying when a particular name is mentioned, family members and attendants assume that the spirits calling for that name have been appeased, and the baby takes the name. This tradition hasn't yet caught on here, as the small numbers of children called Shut, Up, Or, Else, I'll, Batter or You bear out.

For the Nandis of the Great Rift Valley, baby naming takes place in the mother's hut while the men, who have been kept in the dark regarding the baby's sex, wait outside. The mother and attending women call a spirit's name to watch over the baby. The baby is meant to sneeze to indicate that it accepts the name. (Snuff is used to help the sneezing.) The men waiting outside can tell from the women's laughter whether the baby is a girl or a boy. A three-interval laugh means the child's a girl, whereas a four-interval laugh means it's a boy.

In Nandi tradition, the original name that a child receives is not used until a substitute name, birth-related and selected by the mother, is given a few days later. Now this is a fantastic idea. Call the kid whatever you want for a few days and when the euphoria and novelty wear off you can decide whether or not it's worth ruining its life.

These tribes seem to have got naming about right. Wouldn't it be great if the UK, the US and other English-speaking countries could follow suit? Admittedly, sitting around an open fire wearing nothing but a few beads and perhaps a sharp bit of flint to protect your you-know-whats on a piece of common ground outside your council house in the middle of winter waiting for the sacrificial lamb to pop its clogs before you can name your kid isn't that good an idea. But what if you could adapt one of the ancient tribal naming procedures to suit your own lifestyle? Now that would be good.

Imagine the scene. Bonfire night sees you all down the park, donning your latest Adidas bench coat, old pair of Reebok Classics and Burberry scarf (you didn't steal it, but you didn't pay for it either). You've done a lush job of clearing up the dogshit and needles. A little gang's already crowding around a little fire they've started with the help of their older friends, the pre-pubescent pyromaniacs who've been terrorizing your neighbourhood ever since you and your partner knew there was a kid on the way.

A pack of skinny strays that normally roam around at night barking at anything that moves have locked their bull terriers away for once and sit respectfully cross-legged with their backs against the Peugeot they've just jacked from the posh new housing estate the other side of the park. Jimmy Giro, the local tramp who's been stumbling through life shouting at trees and sleeping rough in a snorkel jacket since Jesus was a boy, has a quick swig of super-strength cider, then hollers for silence. The naming ceremony is about to begin.

You and your loved one, clutching your newborn child close to your body so that no one can hear the screams you caused by getting its ears pierced at the age of six days, make your way to the centre of the throng, which by this time is beginning to settle into a respectful hush. It's pitch-black bar the odd flame, which fizzes every time little Dave and his mates from round the block gob into it from impressive distances. Bob the Slob decides against chucking an old aerosol in for a laugh.

The pair of you gently place the kid on a slightly damp pile of old porn mags, sacrifice a couple of cigarettes to the lung god, forget why you're there for a bit and end up naming the child Fiesta-Benson. You all get pissed on Stella, and bar a few arrests for causing a disturbance in a public place, little Fiesta has a name, you've won the admiration of the neighbourhood and everyone can go home happy.

Apart from old Jimmy Giro who's nodded off and is getting set fire to.

Sources
http://www.babyzone.com/
http://www.africaguide.com/
http://library.thinkquestafrica.org/
http://www.runningdeerslonghouse.com/
http://www.mandarintools.com/chinesename.html

Born famous: How to give your child star quality

4

First man: What do you call your daughter?

Second man: Vee.

First man: How come?

Second man: I told my wife I'd name her after you.

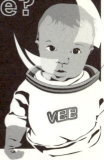

"There's nothing wrong with a bit of nepotism," said the hopeless eldest child of the filthy rich MD of a mega-successful family firm. True. If, however, you're not lucky enough to have been born into a family that makes money for fun, you might want to give your kids some sort of star quality to put them on the right path to fame and riches.

A 40-something woman told us that naming her three children was the most stressful thing she had ever done. She didn't hang around long enough to tell us what names she'd chosen, but what she said probably rings true for most of you reading this book. From a woman's perspective, thinking up a name for a child is another agonizing addition to the list of tortures you have to go through from conception to delivery. Men have no idea how much pressure is put on the bladder, how much the old back hurts and how much being pregnant knackers up your life, from not being to wear any of your favourite designer clothes to fat ankles.

From a woman's point of view, it could be reasonably argued that the man should have no say in naming the child. Isn't that right, girls? What the hell do blokes know, anyway? They're not the ones who've had to suffer the pain, discomfort and all-round hassle for the last nine months. Plus, all their ex-girlfriends had stupid names, and were slags. If you have a daughter, there's no way she's gonna get one of their names, is she? That's right.

The right to have the final say over the naming of your child notwithstanding, one aim for many parents – mothers *and* fathers – is to give their child star quality.

Whether this is actually a good idea is not for us to judge. Instead, this chapter will guide you through the pitfalls inherent in choosing a star name and try and make sense as to why you and countless others may want to imbue your child with some sort of fame-inducing quality by its name alone.

So, mothers, if you've decided that you really want your kid to stand out from the crowd – in other words, you've concluded, and your other half has agreed, that you were right in the first place – you need to utter a load of names out loud, write them down, make sure they don't sound or look awful when coupled with your surname and so forth (see the other chapters for help along these lines – there's advice a-plenty throughout). This is an integral link in the "naming for fame" process chain.

But before that, let us help you get into the right frame of mind. Kick your partner out for a while (if you haven't binned him already, the useless oaf). Tell him to walk the dog or go to the pub or something. Sit down in your favourite chair and arrange the cushions so you're nice and comfy. Turn the telly and hi-fi off. Take a deep breath. Now get up again and make a cup of tea – preferably herbal (peppermint's nice) – and, yeah, go on, grab a chocolate bar, a biscuit or something you know'll make you feel better for now. Come back to your comfy chair, sit in it, take another deep breath and compose yourself.

Now look around the room, and if there's any newspapers, magazines, books, DVDs, CDs or anything with writing on in your line of vision, get up again and hide them from view. You don't want your yet-to-be-born child's name to be in any way influenced by what you've just seen knocking about the living room. If there's a fruit bowl in front of you and your name's Gwyneth, shift it. Oops, too late.

This is where the fun begins. You want your child to be a star, but you don't yet know whether it's gonna be a boy or a girl – unless of course you looked at the scan and cheated, to be organized and all that. Let's presume you don't know the sex of your unborn baby. *SWAYCI* doesn't know, so why should you?

Right. Back to the fame/success thing. You want your child to be a success, and you've got every right to. You may have made a few mistakes along the way – one of which may be the unborn kid (hey, shit happens) – but everyone's entitled to mistake or two, aren't they? (Apart from the government, the police, doctors, lawyers, teachers, football referees and so on.) So, now you've come to terms with being a bit rubbish yourself (no offence), you see naming your offspring as a saving grace. A talking point. Some sort of vicarious kid-driven celebrity status. Whatever your motives may be for wanting your kid to be famous, there are ways and means of achieving it, and the very tip of the fame iceberg is a memorable name. Never forget it. For every Elvis Presley, there are a million Elvis impersonators.

What may be blindingly obvious to *SWAYCI* could be something you've totally overlooked. First, check yourself and your partner out – yes, you've kicked him out for the time being, but you can remember what he's like, can't you? Are either of you famous? If either of you are premiership footballers, Olympic athletes, actors (currently on the telly or in the pictures a lot), politicians (prime minister, cabinet or shadow cabinet only), TV presenters or pop stars (with a top ten hit in the last decade), then, yes, you're famous.

Having appeared on telly in a reality show doesn't make you a star, unless you're Ant and Dec, Davina McCall or Simon Cowell. Especially if you're one of those benefit-fraudster chavs from Rochdale.

If you *are* famous, then congratulations. Enjoy it while it lasts without getting too big-headed and forgetting where you came from, who put you there, blah blah blah. You're in an enviable position, you see: if nothing else, once your fame wanes attention will switch to your child, and you can live out your life through your unusually named son or daughter.

Fame attracts hangers-on, admirers and potential partners, so once you achieve fame yourself, there's every chance you'll have a child somewhere along the bling-plated line. There are many prime examples of having a kid to enhance your profile, such as former *EastEnders* star Jessie Wallace. Knowing that she'd have to leave the programme at least for a while to give birth and look after her first-born, she wanted a way to stay in the public eye. Rather than do something really undignified like fall out of a Soho nightspot at four in the morning (leave that to footballers on compassionate leave), she plumped for the option of giving her daughter a proper rubbish name:

Tallulah Lilac. Remember? Of course you do. It was on the front page of all the tabloids. Oh dear. But to be fair to young Miss Wallace's celebrity mum, there's no chance of TL working in a call centre when she grows up unless she sacks that bobbin's name.

When people ask, in that exasperated way, "What was she thinking about?" the answer is easy. Accentuating her fame by giving her child a crap name. Credit where it's due, though. Ms Wallace served her time at acting school and did a convincing job of playing an overweight, orange-skinned cockney slapper in *EastEnders*, so she probably just about deserves the right.

Obviously, it's easier said than done, becoming famous. Just look at all the thousands of mis-shapen mugs who fail to get to the final stages of *Big Brother*, *Pop Stars*, *Pop Idol*, *The X Factor* et al. In fact, becoming famous legally is damned hard. Don't give up the ghost yet though, or start practising your vocals with a hairbrush in front of the mirror. You don't have to be famous yourself to give your kid a name that's positively oozing star quality. There are a number of techniques you can employ to put your kid on the ladder to success, but to make sure the rungs aren't cracked and full of splinters, heed the following advice.

Work out which famous person's name your own surname most closely resembles. With any luck it'll be an exact letter-for-letter match with the name of a celebrity you actually like. Then simply name your child after them. Your offspring may hate you forever as a result, but what the heck? In a stroke of the registrar's pen you've got a famous kid who needn't do a thing to earn its fame. Brilliant! Free fame: it doesn't come any cheaper than that. If on the other hand your surname is so bizarre that it doesn't match up with anyone famous, just give your child an equally crazy first name, using the relaxation technique described a few paragraphs ago. By the way, another lovely tea is that Echinacea stuff (don't call your kid that though, eh?).

At least if your child has a strange name they won't be forgotten in a hurry. And, as with young Tallulah Lilac, other people won't be in a rush to name their kid after yours. Unless, of course, they want fame by proxy, with you as the proxy.

If you do happen to have a fully fledged famous name yourself, or you're thinking of going down the "add first name to existing surname to copy famous name" route, then you won't mind finding out that there are several thousand people around the world who are in a similar celebrity namesake situation. If you haven't got a famous name yourself, or the idea of deliberately naming your offspring to match an existing famous person fills you with contempt, then you might just enjoy some of the real-life stories *SWAYCI* has put together for you.

You see, some of the stick non-famous people with famous names have to cop for is nothing short of horrendous. We've assembled a few anecdotes to show you what it's like for normal people to have famous names. Reading them might give you a better idea of what you might be letting your newborn in for.

Bill Clinton of Washington, Indiana works as a truck driver, and is among four Bill Clintons in Indiana and 20 in the US. He's a bit of a comedian too: "I tell people that I'm Bill Clinton and I live in Washington, DC – that's Washington in Davies County. I also live in a white house."

And they wonder why so many people in the US have guns. Apparently old Bill didn't even realize he shares his name with a recent ex-president of the US until someone pointed it out to him a few years ago. He cheekily added, "When I tell people my name, they don't believe me. But it doesn't annoy me. I tell them I'm the real Bill Clinton and that other guy is an impostor." Quick, add his name to the party invites. When the elections came around, he apparently voted for himself.

Be very afraid, folks, for he's not alone. Gerald R. Ford of Pittsburg, California voted for himself too. He's always insisted on being called Gerald rather than Gerry because when he was around in World War II he didn't want to be mistaken for a Nazi. Go figure.

His anecdote just goes to show how daft Americans are, as if we needed reminding. "One night when I presented my Diner's Club card to the maître d' on the way into a nice restaurant I was treated very, very well. On the way out I was told, 'Come back soon, Mr Congressman.'"

Whoop-dee-doo.

Ronald McDonald of Rolla, Missouri, was too embarrassed to talk to *SWAYCI*, but his less famous wife was glad to contribute. Apparently the couple knew a man who played the Ronald McDonald clown for the area. The Yanks do have their saving graces, though, to be fair to the burger-munching fools. Mr McDonald and his better half dread using their credit card, as they have to suffer remarks from "You've got to be kidding!" and "Who would name a kid that?" to "How's business?" and "Would you like fries with that, sir?"

Best of all, Mrs McDonald told us, "We used to get phone calls during the night from kids at parties who would ask if they could order some Big Macs. You can laugh at the first few, but after a while it is pretty annoying. Especially at four in the morning."

In fact, *SWAYCI* couldn't shut her up: "Our daughter was crowned homecoming queen at her high school in the middle 1970s, and when they announced her name, they added that she was the daughter of Mr and Mrs Ronald McDonald. There was a loud laughing in part of the crowd and it was an embarrassing moment on an otherwise perfect evening." The couple never eat at McDonald's. Not the famous one anyway.

Marcia Brady of Waterbury, Connecticut kind of missed the point. When *SWAYCI* asked her if she'd ever change her name, she replied, "I would never change it. However, I would change my legs with liposuction. At 50 they don't look that great any more." Thanks for that, mate.

We couldn't find another Madonna Ciccone, but we did get hold of a Sean Penn from Atlanta, Georgia and a Guy Richie from Middlesbrough, UK.

Sean Penn gets a lot of people asking him how Madonna is: "Jeez, they're so stupid! Don't they know that he split up with Madonna, like, years ago"? Of the many namesakes we discovered, he wasn't too bad a guy – for an American. He admits that the real Sean Penn is "a good actor and an excellent director." Mr Penn went on to say, in a more eloquent way than you'd think possible for someone from Atlanta (trust your author – he's been there), "His body of work is varied and I think it shows great range." There's no smoke without fire, though, and the less famous Sean Penn signed off by admitting that "I save magazines where Sean Penn has appeared on the cover. I have several issues of *Rolling Stone*."

On the other hand, Guy Richie, born and bred in the 'Boro (the way locals fondly refer to their home town), is indifferent to the whole thing. A successful banker, Mr Richie played down any name-related fun he might have had since the rise of the director of *Snatch* and *Lock, Stock and Two Smoking Barrels*. "It doesn't bother me in the slightest, nor has it affected my life in any way – good or bad. I've got a good job, a loving wife and two kids. You can't say that for the famous Guy Richie, now can you?"

Er . . . yeah, you sorta can, Guy, to be honest. *SWAYCI* didn't get much change out of Mr Richie, other than to find out that his only memorable namesake moment was when a less than bright receptionist at a hotel once asked him for his surname. When he told her, she quipped, "You don't look much like Lionel."

Back in the good old US of A, however, Colin Powell's less famous namesake provided us with a fine contribution. Apparently Colin – of non-fame fame – even gets letters from people looking for kids missing in action according to his spokesperson, his mother Ann. "The worst part," she said, "is having someone famous who does not pronounce his name the right way."

You've seen just how easy it is to laugh at non-famous people with famous names. As easy, in fact, as it is to laugh at people who'll do anything to be famous. But it's just as simple to be the poor sod on the receiving end of the laughter, whether directed at you or by proxy. So be careful what you do and who you laugh at. In fact, laugh at people only if they can't see or hear you. This works really well when they're on the telly in some *Pop Stars* or other famous-for-fifteen-seconds show they happen to be peddling their tawdry wares on.

If you truly, madly, deeply want your children to be the stars of the show, send them to drama school and prevent them appearing on TV talent shows. You can always use the "I'll show the tabloids your birth certificate" threat as a last resort.

One man's star is of course another man's black hole, so your journey into vicarious fame isn't over yet. One thing you could do to give your child star quality, or at least notoriety, is to get banged up. It doesn't matter what the crime is, although the less grotesque the better. Maybe a touch of tax dodging or forgetfulness when it comes to paying the TV licence. Immediately your kid is famous because of his jailbird parent. It worked for Ronnie O'Sullivan. Look at him: world champion at snooker. Named after his dad too. Excellent move, Mr O'Sullivan. No daft naming trickery for you. *SWAYCI* salutes your efforts to help your son reach the top in his chosen profession and hopes you get out of prison so you can watch him in action.

Alternatively, you could join a rock band and do something controversial involving drugs, groupies and auto-erotic asphyxiation. Better still, get banged up for doing it. Take Ian Brown, former Stone Rose. The cadaverous-faced frontman didn't disgrace himself in the hotel-room-shenanigans arena; he was chucked off the aeroplane before he even got there. After the band split up, Mr Brown got himself into a bit of in-flight bother by allegedly insulting an air stewardess and a pilot, and ended up doing a brief stretch in Strangeways. When his kids realize that he was accused of telling one of the male trolley dollies that he had a shit beard, they'll be happy to be called anything.

Yeah, you're right, imbuing your kid with star quality is pretty damn tricky. You all know deep down that giving your child a ridiculous name is the cheapest and simplest way for it to be the centre of attention, regardless of its talent or lack thereof. That's unless you're totally effing stupid. But as a proud purchaser of *SWAYCI* there's obviously hope for you – and your soon-to-be-born child – yet.

If you're still sitting comfortably, you shouldn't be. Isn't it time you decided on a name? Have you said all the possible names out loud? Have you even written them down? Look out, the other half's back. Quick, hide the book; he need never know that you had to resort to reading it to come up with a name for your imminent arrival. Now look as if you're stressed and need a massage. That's it.

Sources
www.funnynames.com
www.weirdnames.com

Scrabbling around: If you're not religious, why not make up a name?

5

First man: What's your name, mate?

Second man: Horse.

First man: No wonder you've got such a long face.

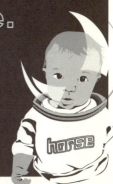

Trace any name back to its roots and you'll find, rather disappointingly, that it's made up. That said, Biblical names at least have some sort of credibility, given that they're so old and generally easy to spell and indeed pronounce. It's no coincidence that the names you hear all the time – Michael, Paul, Peter, Rachel, Mary, Stephen – come from the Bible. Perhaps you should be reading it. Might give you some inspiration.

If you're not a regular Bible reader, a category many of us fall into these days, then maybe it's not the best source of inspiration. Unless you want your new child to be called Loaf, Fish or Burning Bush. If you don't much fancy giving your child a name you've heard before, why not just make something up? Doing so has certain advantages. Inevitably it won't be long before a) other people are following your lead and copying, thus rendering your son or daughter's name normal, or b) your child's old enough to have a group of friends who are happy to rename him or her with some sort of nickname, whether it's lazily adding a default "y," "a" or "oh" to their surname, or something bordering on the surreal.

If your child has a nicknamable surname, you may as well abandon any idea you had of dreaming up a new name right now. A lad called James could reasonably expect to be called Jim, Jimmy or Jamie by his peers or parents, and probably wouldn't mind too much unless he was a fussy, pretentious idiot. So why did a James that we spoke to end up being called Manchild? Simple – his surname was Blanchard and someone once misheard it as Manchild. Obviously, everyone within earshot thought what a great nickname it was, and it stuck. Thus are nicknames born. *SWAYCI*'s author's name can be abbreviated in many ways: Alex, Alec, Ali, Sandy, Eck and so on. But for some reason, most of his peers preferred Lexy. Then, after a post-match pub visit, one of the extended circle of friends (for it is wide) passed comment on Pixie's performance. As with Manchild, it didn't take much persuasion for everyone to start calling him Pixie. Thankfully it didn't stick, although no doubt the legions of *SWAYCI* readers will delight in reminding him of it during the inevitable mass autograph sessions at posh bookshops.

One of the discoveries we made when researching this book was that it wasn't that long ago that almost everyone, certainly in the UK, was named after their mother, father or grandparent. Traditional names such as Albert, Elizabeth, George, Margaret and so on were very much in vogue until as recently as the 1960s. It's only recently that parents have had the bottle/foolhardiness (delete as appropriate) to saddle their children with made-up names.

Even a staunch atheist bibliophobe would know that the name Peter is not only taken from the Bible, but means rock. (Hence the word petrified: to be turned to stone.) But what do all the new-age names mean? Let *SWAYCI* help you with its handy – and snappily titled – List of New-Age Names and What They Might Mean. None of them are made up. No, really.

Aaliyah (#1)
A girl who doesn't tell the truth

Aaliyah (#2)
A boy with a girl's name who doesn't tell the truth

Andrey
Should have been called Andrew or Andrea, but my mum (who can't spell) liked *I'm a Celebrity, Get Me Out of Here*

Apple
A fruit

Benjy
My dad once did a bungee jump

Brooklyn
A district of New York

Caribou
My folks met at a Pixies concert; my twin brother's called Crackity Jones

Clementine
A fruit

Daisy Boo
A rubbish flower / early 90s popstar hybrid

Demornier
My folks are rough as arseholes, but want to sound posh by proxy

Dweezil
Ebeneezer was too good for me (also, see Moon Unit)

Eugenie
My mater is no genius

Fifi Trixibelle
My mother was a bit confused and thought she was naming a show poodle

Georgie
Why not just leave traditional names alone?

Hyacinth
Stinky flower

Indiana
Well, it was good enough for a US state and an intrepid explorer/ archaeologist

Koosha
I still don't know whether I'm a boy, a girl or something you'd fail to identify in a bowl of exotic mixed fruit

Mondeo
Don't name your child after a so-called luxury car

Moon Unit
My old man was as mad as a hatter and probably took lots of mind-altering drugs

Nell Marmalade
Not quite Nell Gwynn, nor the full jar of Robertson's

Peaches
A fruit (plural)

River
Not quite a sea, but bigger than a stream

Rumer
Something you hear about yourself or someone else that might not be true

Satchel
A bag to carry your clothes in

Zowie
A starman waiting in the sky.

With any luck, the names and definitions above will have stimulated you into rational thought about what your kid's name should be and the possible implications for the rest of its life if you make a name up. If as a result of reading our frankly horrific list of names you've decided that you want to give your child a more normal name, then that's fine, honestly. It shows a distinct lack of imagination on your part, but that's nothing to be ashamed of. There are worse things you could do.

A friend of ours has the good fortune to work with kids. She's noticed that the names of the children in her class get more outlandish every year. She told us (and it must be true because she's a teacher and teachers are always right) that when she first taught at a girls' school all the pupils seemed to be called Jennifer, Stephanie or Jessica. Normal names, yes? Now, she tells us, she meets loads of Ashleys and Tiffanys. First, Ashley – surely a boy's name, yes? Second, Tiffany – come on folks, even if you thought you were alone, there didn't seem to be anyone around and you were positive that the beating of your heart was the only sound . . . DON'T CALL YOUR KID TIFFANY! Terrible name, terrible name, terrible, terrible, terrible name. Good Eurovision-style singalong song though.

Popular names change like popular fashion and popular music. At one of the posh dinner parties *SWAYCI* often gets invited to, a Catholic couple with a daughter named Courtney were asked how they had settled upon the name. Thankfully, it wasn't anything to do with Ms Cox or Ms Love. Courtney's mother gave a little sigh and said, "We just liked the way it sounded." Taken at face value, this is the daftest imaginable way to name a child. To make matters worse, Courtney's surname began with a C. We won't reveal her surname in full to preserve her anonymity. It's not her fault, after all. She didn't ask to be called Courtney. If fact, isn't Courtney a traditional West Indian name anyway? I'm sure jazz great Courtney Pine and all-time cricketing legend Courtney Walsh would have something to say about that.

Just engage your brain for five minutes and imagine the moment when someone asks you why you plumped for your kid's name. It ain't rocket science (nor for that matter should it be Moon Unit), but glibly to name your child "because it sounds nice" and bestow upon it alliteration is a total no-no. Guilty guest then added, "I sometimes wish we hadn't called her Courtney because I would like her to have a saint's name." Well perhaps you should have spent a bit longer thinking her name up, eh, darling?

This got us thinking about the way we name our children and the impact these decisions have on them as they grow and develop as people, which of course is the whole idea of this book, so it's lucky this train of thought finally arrived at the brain station. The names Catholics give their children, for example, are meant to reflect their identity in some way. Over the years, the church has encouraged its followers to name its children after holy men and women, with varying degrees of success. The catechism of the Catholic church states, "In Baptism, the Lord's name sanctifies man, and the Christian receives his name in the church. This can be the name of a saint. The patron saint provides a model of charity; we are assured of his intercession." Despite the antiquated gender-specific language, this is intended to apply to the naming of baby girls too.

Some bishops have taken this as a directive that all baptisms and confirmations require saints' names. For Archbishop Michael Sheehan of Santa Fe, New Mexico, a request to baptize a girl Crystal was the last straw – and rightly so. He declined, much to the chagrin of the attendant family. However, the Catholic encyclopaedia acknowledges that "There has never been a time in the history of the church when these injunctions have been strictly attended to." So now you can not only be religious, but also make up a name for your kid without having to live in fear of divine retribution.

Curious as to the extent to which saints' names are given to children, *SWAYCI* went to the US Social Security Administration, which has its own website dedicated to popular babies' names. The database includes all Americans, not just Catholics, but we made several interesting findings. The top ten most popular monikers for boys born in 2002 were all names of saints or biblical figures: Andrew, Christopher, Daniel, Ethan, Jacob, Joseph, Joshua, Matthew, Michael and Nicholas. Although the equivalent list for girls wasn't quite so biblical – Abigail, Alexis, Ashley, Emily, Emma, Hannah, Madison, Olivia, Samantha and Sarah – most of the names could eventually be traced back to the Bible, either as female versions of male names or slight corruptions of biblical originals.

As you move beyond the top 10, the boys' names continue

to have holy influences. Overall, only five of the top 50 – that's 10 percent to all you mathematicians – aren't derived from a saint or holy person, these being the fairly innocuous Austin (let's hope the Austin Powers series of movies had nothing to do with this), Dylan, Hunter, Ryan and Tyler.

On the other hand, only about half of the top 50 girls' names *are* derived from saints. Alyssa, Destiny (let's hope she doesn't plump for the obvious when she has a child), Jasmine, Kayla, Haley, Savannah all make the list with barely a saint or biblical reference among them. Other girls' names in the top 50 include female versions of male names like Brianna (St Brian) and Amanda (St Amand), as well as names of male saints that have become popular for girls, such as Megan (St Meigan) and Jordan (there are six St Jordans, all male). Wonder if *the* Jordan of big boobidoos, no-brain fame knew this?

We aren't suggesting that all these names were chosen because they were saints' names. It's doubtful that many parents who named their little boy Kyle, for example, realize that there was precisely one St Kyle, a Scottish woman.

SWAYCI was also struck by one omission from the top 50. Mary was the undisputed queen of girls' names in this country, ranking number one in popularity from 1880 to 1946. She was briefly overtaken by the name Linda from 1947 to 1953, but then reclaimed the top spot and held it for eight more years. In 1962, Lisa became the most popular name for girls, remaining so until 1970, when

Jennifer took over. In 1972, Mary fell out of the top 10, never to return. Jennifer's reign lasted into the mid-1980s. Since then, Ashley, Jessica and now Emily have held the top spot. But Mary, the queen of all saints, has gone from the top 50.

Ask yourself this question: "Why do we name our children what we do?" Some disgraces, as we've already heard, give their child a name simply because they like the way it sounds; others, thankfully, are more purposeful. A young mother who named her daughter Madison told us that she wanted her daughter to have a gender-neutral name to give her confidence; that way, when she had a job interview, prospective employers would be surprised to see a self-assured young woman enter the room. Good point well made, yes? Unfortunately, her plan may have backfired, as Madison is now pretty much the exclusive territory of girls after Darryl Hannah's mermaid character in the film *Splash* captured the imagination of fish-loving men across America. So not only will the employer know that Madison is a woman, they'll probably be able to guess roughly how old she is.

Hilariously, the name Jordan is in the top 50 for both sexes, although *SWAYCI* predicts a swing towards girls, especially of the chav variety, after the recent exploits of Katie Price. Going back to Madison's mum, regardless of the success or otherwise of her naming strategy, at least she put some thought into it.

As mentioned before, trendy names are like trendy hairstyles, and we all have old photos of ourselves sporting mullets, spikes or fringes that would have Busted running for cover. At least they were temporary, unlike a name. Do you want your child to have the nominal equivalent of a blue rinse all her life? When our children get to an age when they ask why they're called what they are, we owe them a better answer than, "He won Sports Personality of the Year the day before you were born" or "There was this brilliant American sitcom called *Friends* and Phoebe was really funny."

The names we give our children are a reflection of our values and our hopes for what they will become. Some people who value their family name their children after relatives they admire. Some value fame and name their children after well-known athletes or entertainers. Some (thankfully, a small number) have adopted the supremely unfortunate practice of naming their children after things as worthless as products, brands or cable TV networks. These parents have saddled their children with depressingly shallow names such as Lexus, Chanel, Armani, Cartier, Ikea and the unpronounceable Espn (which found its way onto the birth certificates of at least two boys in the US in 2003). The Catholic catechism teaches that the names we are given at baptism are our names for eternity. This doesn't augur well for the young Espns.

"Wait," you say, "if I limit myself to saints and holy people, won't that drastically reduce my range of choices?" In fact, not as much as you might think, and the pool is getting bigger every year. During the papacy of John Paul II, the number of saints increased by almost

500. There are plenty more in the pipeline, too, with over 1,300 people having been beatified.

If you think about it, although the books of the Bible originate from far-flung places like Bethlehem, Jerusalem and Jeddah, many of the names they contain sound pretty western. The reason is simple. The New Testament saints and the holy people from the Hebrew scriptures didn't have the names we know in English. We have simply anglicized them. Andrew the apostle had a Greek name that was pronounced "Ondrayus." So there is nothing to prevent parents translating a saint's name from one language to another. In a wonderful example of a name that doffs its cap to both Catholicism and ethnic heritage, *SWAYCI* uncovered an African-American couple that named their baby son Jiwe, the Swahili word for rock, and a cunning way of naming him after St Peter too.

There are thousands of grandiose-sounding ethnic names that actually mean something knocking about around the world. Why make a name up when you could pick one of these?

BOYS

African
Adio (righteous), Daudi (beloved), Zuberi (strong)

Chinese
Chen (great), Jun (truth), Li (strength)

Greek
Cyril (lord), Demetrius (lover of earth)

Hindu
Dlnendra (the god of sky), Firoz (winner)

Irish
Aidan (warm), Connor (much desired), Riordan (minstrel)

Native American
Elsu (falcon in flight), Hula (eagle), Nigan (leading the way)

GIRLS

African
Jaha (dignity), Kasinda (born after twins)

Chinese
An (peace), Lin Lin (cheerful), Hua (flower)

Greek
Althea (healer), Sophia (wisdom), Zoë (life)

Hispanic
Lareina (the queen), Alva (pure)

Irish
Deirdre (fear), Maeve (delicate), Kelly (female soldier)

Japanese
Akahana (red flower), Kazu (obedient)

Native American
Kaya (older sister), Hialeah (beautiful pasture).

Which leads us nicely to a few questions you should ask yourself – strictly on a spiritual level – before you attach a name to your new kid:

[✓] **When naming my child, what is the most important thing to take into consideration?**

[✓] **If I had to choose my own name, what would I pick and why?**

[✓] **Do I owe it to my child to give it a name that reflects my religious values and heritage?**

[✓] **Am I named after a saint or biblical figure?**

[✓] **Do I have any sort of a relationship with a saint or biblical figure that I consider my patron?**

[✓] **Should I choose a saint's name over a secular one even if I'm not realistically going to take time to learn about this saint and ask him or her to pray for my child on a regular basis?**

Ask yourself these questions and you'll have a head start on other soon-to-be parents. With the answers fresh in your mind, get yourself a pen and paper. This next bit is for ladies only, so men, off you go and make your missus a brew. She deserves it. For the only time in your life, she's the one who looks most like a darts player.

Start writing down your favourite names. Ideally, you'd be doing this somewhere in the middle of your pregnancy. You don't even need to tell your partner if you don't want to. Kick off with first names. Next, move on to middle names (if you want one, that is – it's not compulsory), and list them separately. You'll probably choose many of the names purely because you like them, but some may remind you of a special friend or family member. Now start combining the first and middle names. Next, add your last name. It may sound obvious, but some people forget; you'll only realize how important it is when you get to the list of names at the end of the chapter.

Some first and middle names go brilliantly together, like peppermint tea and a bar of chocolate (not that that's a naming suggestion, you understand), but when you add the last name it just doesn't work. Write the names out in full to see how they look, and then read them aloud to hear how they sound. This is better done alone; if nothing else, it gives you a chance to use daft voices.

Now rate the names. Write down all the options and combinations (try to keep it under 50 or it becomes too difficult to manage), and then eliminate names one at a time. When you have your top ten, put the list away.

Revisit it a few weeks later. You'll be surprised how your feelings may have changed. Make copies of your list and take it along when you visit friends, family, business associates, total strangers, whoever, so you can ask their opinions. Get them to tell you what they *really* think. By the way, you still need to take what they say with a pinch of salt. It's your baby after all. When Aunt Sadie starts pushing for Mildred Dorothy, which just happens to be her great-grandmother's name, by all means give her the time of day. Just keep repeating "I'm choosing my baby's name, I'm choosing my baby's name, I'm choosing my baby's name" to yourself in your head.

You've come a long way now, and you've learnt that there's a lot of pressure involved in choosing a name – although perhaps not as much as your unborn child is putting on your bladder right now. A name is one of the first things people learn about a child, and it will be a part of them for the rest of their life.

As we've seen, naming your newborn is a daunting process, but it can also be a laugh. Some couples argue about the name right up to the moment when they have to sign the birth certificate. Others think of a name and find they both love the way it sounds. There are probably as many ways to pick a name as there are names.

Has he made that brew yet, or what? Shout him in; he'll like the next bit. Here's a few cautionary tales to help you on your way to giving your kid the ideal name.

Ardis and Yaffle

My husband and I named our second child Ardis Daphne. Ardis is my mother's maiden name and Daphne is one of the characters in *Scooby Doo*. Our young son, Yaffle, used to watch it all the time. We named him after Professor Yaffle, the wise carved wooden bookend from *Bagpuss*.

Ethel Morris, Hull

Cassandra

I was six months' pregnant during a trip to Cyprus for a wedding, and there was a large span of time when I couldn't feel the baby move. My doctor kept reassuring me I was walking so much that I was rocking the baby to sleep. On the flight home, still nervous, I decided to try to relax by finishing my Danielle Steel novel. Just as I started reading, the baby kicked. The main character in the book is Cassandra, which is now our daughter's name. And no, she looks nothing like the one out of Only Fools and Horses, *thank God!*

Jane Finch, Luton

Finn

We both come from a very strong Irish background, and we definitely wanted the heritage to live on. I remembered reading the Celtic legend of Finn McCool as a kid. Not only was this the coolest name I'd ever heard, it also transpired that Finn was a giant who did great deeds – an all-round top bloke. So my son's name was chosen 20 years before he actually arrived.

Bernie Gallagher, Sheffield

Gary

Growing up in Birmingham in the late 1970s and early 1980s, I was a massive Villa fan. My walls were plastered with pictures of the beautiful blond bombshell Gary Shaw. I knew that if I ever had a son, there was only one name for him.

Stephanie Blow, Sutton Coldfield

Jemuel

We had set a precedent by calling our first son Solomon, so we didn't want to go down the Michael or Patrick route for our second. Sharon's favourite book is *To Kill a Mockingbird*, which features a character called Jem Finch. We liked the name but knew people would think it was short for Jeremy or Jeremiah, neither of which are good school playground names. We looked in the Old Testament and found a peripheral character called Jemuel, who was the son of Simeon, who was the son of Jacob. That clinched it for us. After all this hard work, Jem broke onto the charts two months later as a female singer-songwriter! Ho hum.

Joel Civico, Epping

Liam and Declan

Both our sons got their names from my husband and I going to the pictures. We picked the name Liam (Neeson, just in case of confusion) for our first boy after watching *Rob Roy* when I was pregnant. Our second son, Declan, was named after Richard Gere's character in **The Jackal**, not after the Geordie titch out of Ant and Dec.

Sharon McMahon, Middlesbrough

Noah James

I've always had a huge crush on musician and actor Rick Springfield. My first son was named after my father, but my second son, Noah James, was named after two of Rick's screen characters. My husband wouldn't let me call him Rick, so I got creative!

Kathryn Collins, Rutherglen

Sammy

When I was pregnant, my husband Bob and I were getting sick of everyone asking us what names we had in mind. So Bob made up names as a joke: XTC for a girl and Zamfir for a boy. I was so sure we were having a boy that I started calling the baby Zammy. When my doctor confirmed that it was a boy, Zammy stuck. Of course, we didn't want our son going through life having to explain all that every time he met someone new, so Sammy was the next best thing. It's a shame some rock stars and actors don't think that way!

Debbie Craig, Glasgow

ZANE

WHEN WE GOT TOGETHER WITH SOME FRIENDS WHO HAD JUST NAMED THEIR BABY BOY JACOB, I TOLD THE NEW MOTHER THAT I REALLY LIKED THE NAME. HER MOTHER-IN-LAW, WHO WAS ALSO THERE, ADDED, "THANK GOODNESS THEY DECIDED TO GO WITH JACOB. THEIR OTHER CHOICE WAS ZANE. CAN YOU BELIEVE IT? WHAT AN AWFUL NAME!" MY HUSBAND AND I LOOKED AT EACH OTHER AND LATER AGREED THAT ZANE WAS EXACTLY THE NAME WE WANTED. I'M SURE MY FRIEND'S MOTHER-IN-LAW WAS APPALLED WHEN

SHE GOT THE BABY ANNOUNCEMENT! BUT WHO GIVES A SHIT WHAT SHE THINKS ANYWAY? ALSO, HOW COOL IS ZANE LOWE?

Jennifer Brown, Huddersfield

That's enough of listening to people you've never met. You'll have noticed that for some parents, the perfect name is as close as their telly or local multiplex. Prime-time shows are rife with characters whose monikers might strike a chord: Sharon, Frank, Den, Kat, Mo and so on. And there are lots of promising names among actors too: Gwyneth (why did you call your kid Apple, darling? Are you mad?), Halle (apparently not named after Manchester's famous orchestra) and Bruce.

One current trend is to name kids after places. We all know about Brooklyn Beckham (lucky he wasn't conceived in Peckham, eh?), but such names as Asia, Cheyenne, China, Dakota, India and Savannah are all gaining in popularity. Americans seem to like using surnames as first names, which we think is crazy. Girls around the country are being saddled with Bentley, Coleman and Ridgely, and boys with Johnson and Jackson.

Still no idea, or are you getting there? If you've read this far and you're still struggling, it's not the end of the world. At least you've been sensible and not rushed into something you'll regret later. We're here to help you avoid any future embarrassment, so how about trying out this simple random made-up name generator.

Your first two letters must be a vowel and a consonant from your favourite TV show. The order you put them in doesn't matter (for example, if you choose EastEnders, you can pick a or e with s, t, n, d or r). The next letter has to be the third letter of your mother's maiden name. (If you don't know who your mother is, don't worry, just pick your favourite letter. Better still, the third letter of what you'd like your mother's maiden name to have been.) If you like the sound of your three-letter concoction, stop now. If not, read on.

OK, letter four must be the second letter of your favourite colour, but only if you haven't now generated a name with three consecutive consonants, because that would be really stupid, self-defeating and totally against *SWAYCI*'s ethos. If you have, just pick any vowel from your favourite colour. The beauty of this name generator is that like a contortionist credit-card salesperson, it has built-in flexibility.

Right. Now your new kid's name-to-be is four letters long. If you're happy and you know it, clap your hands. If it makes you feel better. Otherwise, carry on for letter number five. (We'll talk about numbers as names later. For now, just accept that letter number five is a letter and not a number, in the same way that the number five has only four letters, the word palindrome isn't a palindrome, and monosyllabic has five syllables.) Still awake? Good. Confused? Even better.

So, you've picked four letters and you're still not happy. Right then, try adding the last letter of your first girlfriend or boyfriend's surname. Nobody ever forgets that. Relationships come and go, but you'll always remember your first by first name and surname. Test yourself. However much you try, you'll never be able to think of your first boyf/girlf's first name without the sound of their surname popping up in your mind half a second later.

Your kid now has a unique five-letter name. Surely that's enough letters. No? OK, in that case the first vowel of the name of your favourite football team needs to go next. Don't worry if you don't follow football, just think of a friend who does and use their team. If you don't know who they support, shame on you. You can't be a true friend. If all else fails, look at the sports section, pick a team whose name you like and take a vowel from it. (By the way, QPR means Queens Park Rangers.)

So, there's a six-letter name lurking that's got your kid's name written on it, as it were. Still not happy? OK. Think about the teacher you hated most at school. Letter seven is the first letter of their name. (If you never went to school, use the first letter of the truancy officer's surname or the first letter in the registration of the first car you nicked. In fact, why not just hand the kid over the moment it's born. Someone more worthy will happily bring it up, and it will never need know Burberry exists.)

To round up this chapter, here's a list of names that may look acceptable at first glance, but sound preposterous when you read them out. You never know, you might have wanted to use one of them yourself.

Aaron C. Reskew
Al Beback
Alf Abett
Amos Skittow
Amy Stake
Andy Tover
Ann Chovie
Ann Tandek
Ann Tenor
Anna Dapter
Anna Gram
Anna Kronism
Anna Rack
Anna Reksic
Anne Kersaway
Anne Tellope
Annette Kurtain
Annie Versary
Archie Pelagow
Arnie Dadrink
Arthur Ritus
Avery Niceman
Ben Dinroad
Bertha de Bluze
Betty Diddent
Brandon Eyon
Bill Dersyard
Briony Points
Brooke Ennail
Barbara Seville
Barry Cuwder

Barry O'Reafe
Baxter D. Wall
Bea Keeper
Ben Arner
Carmen Geditt
Carrie-Ann Crowe
Carrie Dowt
Carrie Micote
Carrie Oakey
Carrie R. Baggs
Carrie Smattick
Celia Fate
Chris P. Duck
Chris Spackett
Christopher Wave
Claire Voyant
Cody Pendant
Colin Allcarrs
Colin Derr
Constance Noring
Crispin Even
Crystal Chandra Lear
Curtis E. Carr
Cy Burnett
Cy Kocess
Dan Gerous
Dan Glebitts
Dan Gling
Dee Lyted
Dee Zaster
Denise R. Nobbly

Dennis Elbow
Drew Peacock
Earl E. Bird
Enid Adrink
Erica Nurney
Ed Banger
Ed Overeels
Ed Turner
Edina Cloud
Eileen Dover
Ella Mentry
Ella Vator
Ellie Gant
Ellie Kopter
Euan Huzarmy
Eva Brick
Eva Sye
Evan Elpuss
Evan Nowes
Evan Sabove
Evan Tually
Eve Alminds
Eve Apporate
Eve Ninall
Faye McAdemey
Faye Derway
Faye Kinitt
Faye Sake
Faye Slift
Fiona Friend
Flo Tinaway

Flora Bunder
Freda Innocent
Freda Livery
Freda Gogh
Fleur Tashuss
Fran Tick
Gary Oakey
Gill Tedd
Grace Quirrel
Gunther Lunch
Hal Hitosis
Heidi Valuables
Helen Back
Helen Highwater
Herb Altey
Howard Ino
Honour Mission
Hugh Dunnitt
Hugo First
Hugo Tobed
Ian de Dark
Ian de Deepend
Ian O'Sphere
Ida Down
Isabel Ringing
Isla Bebach
Isla Blidge
Isla White
Jack Pott
Jean Poole
Jenna Rossity

Jim Nastic	Lou Bricant
Jim Pansey	Lou Cowt
Joanna Dance	Lou Decruss
Joe King	Lou Natic
Joel Rebocks	Lou Pole
Juan Manband	Lou Scannon
Juan Moment	Lou Smorralls
Juan Mortyme	Lucy Lastik
Julie Thaliteon	Luke Over
Jurgen Ergeditt	Madge Ority
Justin Case	Major Jump
Justin Hale	Major Luke
Justin Nuth	Mal Adjusted
Justin Thyme	Mal Twiskie
Kathy Dralspire	Mal Odruss
Kerry Dowt	Malcolm Tent
Kerry Seen	Mandy Lifeboats
Klaus Shave	Marcus Absent
Kurt Ainring	Marie Inhaste
Lance Lyde	Marsha Mallow
Lars Torders	Matt Ress
Laura Norder	Matt Tromeny
Leah Tard	Megan Bacon
Lee King	Mel Lowe
Lee Vitout	Mel O'Dramer
Lena Meete	Natalie Drest
Les Ismorr	Neil Downe
Lindsay Doyle	Neil Ethere
Lois Bidder	Nick Rofillia
Lois Team	Noah Vale
Lola Beedow	Nora Bone
Lorna Tenis	Oliver de Place

Oliver Sudden
Ophelia Paine
Orson Cart
Orson Ounds
Owen Monie
Paige Turner
Pat Taytow
Pat Tranage
Paul Barer
Penny Chew
Penny Foram
Penny Less
Penny Sillen
Percy Cute
Percy Veer
Perry Scope
Perry Winkel
Pete Zahutt
Phil Itafiche
Phil Itten
Phil Maglassop
Phil McAvity
Philippa Bucket
Phylis Stein
Ray Deator
Ray Ling
Ray Sersharpe
Ray Sleader
Rick O'Shea
Ron Devue
Robin Banks
Robin Emblind

Roland Butter
Rory Motion
Rosa Teeth
Ross Trum
Rowan Bote
Ruby Konn
Rudi Mentry
Russell Sprout
Sadie Word
Sally Mander
Sam Oswer
Sam Widge
Sarah Bellam
Scott Chegg
Seymour Flesh
Sheila Blidge
Shirley Knott
Sir Kit Breaker
Stan Doffich
Stan Dupp
Steve Adore
Sue Dunome
Sue Permann
Sue Purvisor
Sue Ridgepipe
Tania Hyde
Teresa Crowd
Teresa Green
Terry Cottar
Terry Fie
Tia Dropps
Titus Addrum

Tom Bowler
Val Haller
Wanda Doff
Wanda Phull
Warren Peece
Wat Apistle

Wayne Dropp
Will Ting
Willie Belong
Wilma Cargo
Xavier Money
Xavier Self

Some names just don't go together. Even made-up ones.

Sources
http://www.ssa.gov/OACT/babynames/

Team player: If the name fits, wear it on your football shirt

6

Why do they call United's new goalkeeper Dracula?

'Cos he's afraid of crosses!

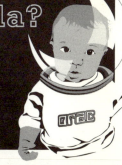

If there's one thing Brazil is better at than churning out world-class footballers, it's churning out fantastic footballers' names. As if conceived by romantic poets, they evoke passion, decadence and euphoria:

Ronaldinho!
Edhinho!
Pele!
Ronaldo!
Juninho!
Socrates!

If they'd been born in the UK they'd have been Ronny, Eddy, Pete, Ron, Jim and Steve.

There's a certain *je ne sais quoi* to foreign footballers' names that you just don't get at home. Consider the names of some of the most gifted British footballers of all time – George Best, Stanley Matthews, Duncan Edwards, Bobby Charlton, Bryan Robson (ooh careful, Bryan with a *y* – eccentric), Rodney Marsh, Stan Bowles, Francis Lee (which would have been a bit classy had it not fallen foul of the "both names are surnames" rule). This lot sound as if their parents were asleep when they named them, or at least in a state of mild lethargy. Which perhaps explains why the defenders who had to face them displayed similar tendencies.

You have to be just as careful when naming footballers as you would normal people. Footballers' names, you see, work properly only in their correct context and in their purest form. Beware the temptation of naming your child after a footballer. It's more of a minefield than a football field.

A Sunday league referee from a modest town in the south of England loved the 1970 Brazil World Cup–winning side so much that he named his first boy Jairzinho. Now some names don't travel beyond Copacabana. Jairzinho sounds wonderful as a name for a sublimely talented Brazilian footballer, but it doesn't trip off the tongue in a Colchester playground. Poor old Essex Jairzinho got so fed up having the mickey (wonder if they say *michel* in France or *miguel* in Spain?) taken out of him by his schoolmates, not least for his distinctly average footballing abilities, that he now goes by the name of Anthony. Apparently he once owned a clockwork orange.

There are loads more true stories – and many apocryphal ones – about club-footed kids being named after top footballers and failing to live up to the hype. It's sad, really, but the blame lies solely at the similarly untalented feet of the parents. You.

We can learn a lot from the way the Brazilians name their footballers. It's simple: all you do is give your kid a really long name, maybe with two or more middle names, see if they come to anything on a football pitch, and then if they're any cop change the name. Don't saddle the poor kid with a name he's never going to live up to in a month of Saturdays before he's even made that intelligent, technically gifted head-first slide from the womb all the way into the safe hands of the midwife, who was nicely positioned on the edge of the box to make the save.

Many Brazilian footballers adopt the names of outstanding international players from the past. Real Madrid's Ronaldo was a big fan of the 1960s São Paulo strike partnership of brothers Ron and Aldo De Silva, so he renamed himself as a neat combination of the two. Apparently Brazilian footballers also take their names from those of famous film stars and singers, but not the greatest footballer of all. Edson Arantes do Nascimento: now that's what you call a name. His footballing nickname? Not Eddy, Aran or Mento. Pele.

For the record, he was the most famous footballer of his generation, and arguably of all time. He joined his local club, Santos, in 1956, and stayed there until he retired in 1974, helping his side to nine league titles in 18 years. He played for the winning side in the World Cup, football's biggest prize, three times: a feat unsurpassed by anyone before or since.

What a great nickname, eh? But it's only great because he was half decent at football and could score the odd goal (over a thousand, as it happens). Don't make the mistake of giving your kid an exotic footballer's name until he's a brilliant footballer. If he's happier with a golf club, dart or baseball bat in his hand, so be it. It's not your fault he ended up a football hooligan.

Imagine Pele was playing today. He'd have sports shops all over the world ruing their luck. Four letters at a pound a throw. If only he'd kept his original name.

Many theories have been put forward as to how Pele got his footballing nickname. We have two favourites. One: his mates were a bit thick and couldn't pronounce his real name properly.

Two: by the time his team-mates had shouted out his name so he'd pass them the ball, he'd already dribbled past nine of the opposition and buried it in the back of the net. The real reason, of course, is that Pele means, well, er . . . absolutely nothing. Even the great man himself can't remember how and why he ended up as Pele.

Brazilians have got it right on the naming front, that's for sure. Even in formal situations, they use first names. Abbreviated nicknames are equally acceptable. Imagine if that applied to the UK. You could go right up to Prince Charles, bold as brass, and give it, "All right, Chaz?" or "How's it going, Charlie?" without risking a lengthy stint at her Majesty's pleasure. Forget the Prime Minister bit; Tony Blair would be Ant, Tone or just T if he was feeling particularly down with the homies. Yo. Not that you'd see either of them within kicking distance of some of the UK's most competitive Sunday football league teams: London's Hackney Marshes or Manchester's Hough End, say.

There's plenty of lads who have built their amateur football reputations on having similar names to famous footballers. Young Rob Marsh from Pelsall got his debut in the Walsall and district Sunday league because he sounded like a footballer. Statistically speaking, the plainer the name, the better the player in UK football. It's no surprise that on those hundreds of muddy, sloping Sunday morning pitches, 33 percent of the players are called Dave, 33 percent Steve and 33 percent Pete. What about the remaining 1 percent? A motley assortment of monosyllabic surnames with the letter y tacked on the end, that's what.

To imbue our legendary footballers with some fragment of foreign flair, *SWAYCI* has taken the liberty of renaming some of the greatest British footballers of all time. Recognize any of these flamboyantly named fellas?

Nobi Schteelesch
Roberto Moorio
Giorgio Besti
Jean Charltz
Keni D'Alglicio
Roberto Charltioni
Patrice Jeninz

Even with our foreign-sounding embellishments, these guys' names aren't a patchio on some of the world greats. Mention them in the same breath as the names of some of the most gifted players from around the world and UK footballers sound like a bunch of benevolent grandads.

The names Dino Zoff, Franco Baresi and Paulo Maldini suit sharply dressed gangsters meeting in a swanky New York restaurant to eat spaghetti and swear their way through reminiscences of the mooks they've pistol-whipped or strangled with telephone wire. Meanwhile our dull old bunch of Georges, Franks and Gordons sit in their old people's home sharing out the Werthers Originals as they politely discuss the virtues of *Fly Fishing* by J. R. Hartley.

Like it or not, even the Germans have more spectacular footballers' names than we do. Oh ja. Take the up-first, towel-down trio Franz Beckenbauer (the only man to have won the World Cup as both player and manager), Gerd

Muller (aka Der Bomber/Der Dicker = the bomber/the fat man) and Sepp Maier (the long-shorted, big-gloved inspiration for three decades of clowns and porn stars). Annoying, isn't it, knowing your bitterest rivals will always have the upper hand?

Although to bring them down a peg or two, the Germans also have in their midst the ex-Celtic players Schidt and Schiedt (pronounced with a silent d) and England's 1996 European Championship nemesis, the aptly-named Stefan Kuntz. Middlesbrough once had Uwe Fuchs (work the pronunciation out for yourself) on its books and was rumoured to be in the running for the aforementioned Kuntz. What a team sheet that would have been. The other nine wouldn't have had a look-in. No Brazilian-sounding first names could have saved their schnitzel.

On the subject of first names, what were Herr and Frau Schoen doing when they named their son – who went on to become manager of West Germany – Helmut? Helmut Schoen – get it? Excuse me, mate, your fly's down.

Some of you may be struggling with the pronunciations here, but you're in estimable company. It's no secret that British football commentators have fallen foul of mispronunciation more times than they've had hot clichés. The 1990 World Cup Golden Boot winner Toto Schillaci started off the group stage as Shillarkee, became Shillatzee when he'd reached the semis and ended up Skillatchee (the closest approximation to the correct pronunciation) by the time Italy had sewn up the final.

Hasan Sas of Turkey endured a similar moniker metamorphosis during the World Cup in 2002. He kicked off as dull old baldy Hasan Sas, but after his side won a couple of games he became Hasan Sash, and his head became a little shinier. The semi-final came around and he was now Hashan Sash, with a head like a beige pool ball. For the third and fourth play-off matches, the commentator took out his false teeth and rechristened him Hashan Shash. By this point, the shininess of his head was being blamed for everything from SARS to international terrorism.

Closer to home, the deified ex–Manchester United striker and kung fu expert Eric Cantona (Can-ton-ah) was plain old Eric Can-tone-a while at glum Hovis-eating, whippet-breeding Yorkshire outfits Leeds United and Sheffield Wednesday. As a teenager in the 1980s, this author was particularly taken with the Spanish international Lopez Ufarte (pronounced You Farty). Anyone reading *SWAYCI* who doesn't find farts funny, please put the book down now and leave it for someone with a sense of humour.

West London side QPR once had the fearsome strike pairing Shittu and Doudou. Yes, readers, they were crap, but at least their first names didn't fan the flames. Unlike West Brom's Swiss fullback Bernt Haas. It's just a shame none of them ever played for Arsenal.

The next trio could have played for Arsenal ladies' team and got away with it. Marian Pahars, Karel Poborski and Pegguy Arphexad are just three examples of professional footballers whose parents can't have had the foggiest idea about British naming conventions. Or perhaps they'd always wanted daughters?

Stability Unit, Black Sunday and Rhoo are just some of the nicknames fans have given to South Africa's top footballers to reflect their skills. (Wouldn't it be good if some players had no names whatsoever, to reflect their lack of skills?) Orlando Pirates' Stability Unit, incidentally, got his nickname because of his ability to marshal his side's defence. And his real name? Plain old Gavin Lane. There's probably fifty Gavin Lanes playing Sunday football in the UK right now, all of whom answer to either Gav or Laney.

Black Sunday, real name Musasa, earned his nickname by scoring goals that helped his then club TP Mazembe knock opponents Chiefs (to which he later transferred) out of an important cup competition. Sometimes, however, the nickname given to a player has nothing to do with his appearance or skill level. Lucas Radebe was dubbed Rhoo because of the way the name echoes around a stadium when thousands of fans are chanting it at once. Hirsute South African centre-half Mark Fish is referred to as Fisssssssssssssshhhhhhh for similar reasons. (Apparently he had previously complained to team officials because fans were calling him Fish and Chips.) Lanky Estonian goalkeeper Mart Poom's surname undergoes similar treatment from his ardent supporters.

Former Bafana Bafana midfielder John Moshoeu is universally known as Shoes. Like Pele, he got the nickname as a child and can't remember how. Mmm . . .

maybe something to do with the second syllable of your surname, mate?

Kaizer Chiefs fan Maloko Lichaba has a theory: "Usually one or two people mention a nickname in a pub or a shebeen and fans familiarize themselves with that name. They go to the stadium and start chanting that name and the next thing you know is that the newspapers use the name and it stays."

Most of the names in the African league are original and relate to players' physical appearance or style of play, but a few derive from TV shows or films. Some players are even named after racehorses. In the 1970s, Kansas Chiefs had a speedy winger, Leonard Likoebe, who acquired the nickname Wagga Wagga from a horse that won a July handicap in Durban. In the UK, Man City and England player Colin Bell was also named after a race horse, Nijinski. To the chagrin of Man United fans, neither end at the new City of Manchester Stadium was named after City's legendary player. Think about it. Staying in the UK, Lincoln City in the late 1950s had a defender called Ray Long who was over six feet tall. The same team boasted a five foot four winger called David Short.

Nowadays, of course, British-based sides tend to employ foreign coaches to tell them what to do. Football being football, a lot of these blokes will have been sacked by the time you read this, but at the time of writing Chelsea had Mourinho, Spurs had Santini and Arsenal had Wenger. Even Dario Gradi was still Crewe Alexandra boss. Having a foreign boss at the helm instantly imbued these clubs with that extra bit of glamour. Even so, anyone with a passing interest in football will know that the London clubs have always fancied themselves as a bit special, but when it comes down to it, it's the Midlands and the north that have won the European cups under Brian, Tony, Alex and Bob.

Finally, let's not forget that Brazilian football owes everything to the mundanely named Charles Miller, the son of a Scottish rail worker who lived in São Paulo. Legend has it that it was he who took the first footballs to Brazil in 1894 from his school in Southampton. If only he'd done what Roger Miller of Cameroon did a hundred years later and change his name to Milla to make it sound more exotic, then he might have got a game.

Sources
http://www.football365.com
http://www.zoofootball.com
http://www.safc.com
http://newswww.bbc.net.uk/sport1/hi/football/africa/3354137.stm

My future's so bright, I gotta wear shades: The phuture of naming

7

Knock knock.
Who's there?
Doctor.
Doctor Who?

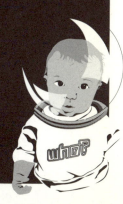

You're not getting any younger, your biological clock's ticking away and your kid's ready to pop out into an age when mobile phones are the size of a pinhead and can do everything except the dishes. So far, you've read about all sorts of methods and techniques to choose a decent name for your offspring. You've heard about biblical names, tribal names and made-up names, but what's in store for the next generation? How are your kids going to decide what to call their children? What names will they come up with, and what circumstances will influence *their* choices?

The future of naming is an uncertain one, but *SWAYCI* has jumped into its Tardis, stared into its crystal ball and left its tea leaves in the bottom of its cup to predict what may happen when it's time for your children to start worrying in the same way that you are right now. Consider this: one direction that parents of the digital age could take is to name their kids after famous robots. And why not? Whatever era you happen to be around in, the past always has appeal. By the time your kids are old enough to start stressing about what they're going to call their own children, all the names listed below will be ancient, yet they come from various people's visions of the future. Clever, eh?

Take a look at these android names from TV and the movies as a little guide to the robot names currently available for exploitation. (Our thanks to the Podster website for permission to borrow their list.)

Able
(Red Dwarf)

Adam
(The Outer Limits)

Alan Talbot
(The Twilight Zone)

Alice in Wonderland
(Star Trek)

Alice Series
(Star Trek)

Alicia
(The Outer Limits)

Alicia
(The Twilight Zone)

Alpha One
(The Flash)

Alpha 5
(Mighty Morphin Power Rangers)

Andrea
(Star Trek)

Android Lloyd Wellington III
(Homeboys in Outer Space)

Andromus
(Galactica 1980)

Andromidus
(Galactica 1980)

Andy
(Luna)

Andy
(Quark)

A.N.G.I.E.
(Sliders)

Ani
(Mercy Point)

April
(Buffy the Vampire Slayer)

Archie
(Red Dwarf)

Argonauts
(Children of the Dog Star)

Ariana
(Logan's Run)

Automated Personnel Units
(Star Trek: Voyager)

Autons
(Doctor Who)

Avalon
(Blake's 7)

Bartender
(Omega Doom)

Battle Droids
(Star Wars I, IV, V, VI)

Batty, Roy
(a replicant)
(Blade Runner)

Bishop
(Aliens, Alien3)

B.O.B.
(The Black Hole)

Bolen, John
(Class of 1999 II: The Substitute)

Borgraf, R.
(Robots)

Box
(Logan's Run)

Bubo
(Clash of the Titans)

Call, Annallee
(Alien Resurrection)

Captain S.T.A.R.
(The Black Hole)

Cassandra
(Android)

Chalmers
(Spacehunter: Adventures in the Forbidden Zone)

Chani
(Devil Girl from Mars)

Chatzpe
(Mastermind)

Clean Up Droids
(Star Wars I, IV, V, VI)

Clickers
(Creation of the Humanoids)

Confessional
(Sleeper)

Coppelia
(Dr Coppelius)

Crow
(Mystery Science Theater 3000: The Movie)

C-3PO
(Star Wars I, IV, V, VI)

Cylons
(Battlestar Galactica, Conquest of the Earth)

Dagget
(Battlestar Galactica, Conquest of the Earth)

Daneel Olivaw, R.
(Robots)

Danner
(Circuitry Man, Plughead Rewired: Circuitry Man II)

Daryl
(D.A.R.Y.L.)

Data
(Star Trek: First Contact, Generations, Insurrection)

David
(A.I.: Artificial Intelligence)

Deco, Artie
(Hardware Wars)

Destroyer Droids
(Star Wars I, IV, V, VI)

Dewey
(Silent Running)

Droids
(Omega Doom)

ED-209
(Robocop)

Electric Servant
(The Electric Servant)

Elle
(Starcrash)

Enforcer Drone
(Spaced Invaders)

Eve
(Eve of Destruction)

Evolver
(Evolver)

Fem-Bot
(Austin Powers 2: The Spy Who Shagged Me)

4-Q-2
(Hardware Wars)

Galaxina
(Galaxina)

Gigolo Joe
(A.I.: Artificial Intelligence)

Girl Bombs
(Dr Goldfoot and the Girl Bombs)

Giskard, R.
(Robots)

G9 iPerson
(Robot Stories)

Gog
(Gog)

Golddigger
(Robot in the Family)

Golem Robots
(Starcrash)

Gort
(The Day the Earth Stood Still, Dr Satan's Robot, The Mysterious Dr Satan)

Great One, The
(Robot Monster)

Gunslinger
(Westworld)

Gypsy
(Mystery Science Theater 3000: The Movie)

Head, The
(Omega Doom)

Hector
(Saturn 3)

Hel
(Metropolis)

Helle
(Starcrash)

Hermes
(The Spaceman and King Arthur)

Huey
(Silent Running)

Interrogation Droids
(Star Wars I, IV, V, VI)

Jane, R.
(Robots)

Jay Seven
(Navigatori dello Spazio)

Jinx
(Space Camp)

John
(Planeta Burg)

Johnny Five aka Number 5
(Short Circuit, Short Circuit 2)

J269
(Automatic)

K-9
(Doctor Who)

Karlo
(The Lost Planet)

Klyton
(Robot Holocaust)

Kragus
(Creation of the Humanoids)

Kronos
(Kronos)

Kryten
(Red Dwarf)

L
(Starcrash)

Lagan
(a clicker) (Creation of the Humanoids)

Leon
(a replicant) (Blade Runner)

Lesli
(The Dark Side of the Moon)

Little Kyser
(a replicant) (Blade Runner)

Louie
(Silent Running)

Lucifer
(a Cylon) (Battlestar Galactica, Conquest of the Earth)

Magnificent Major
(The Magnificent Major)

Magog
(Gog)

Maintenance Droids
(Star Wars I, IV, V, VI)

Mandroid
(Mandroid)

Mark
(a clicker) (Creation of the Humanoids)

Mark 13
(Hardware)

Marvin
(The Hitch Hiker's Guide to the Galaxy)

M.A.X.
(Encounter in the Third Dimension)

Max 404
(Android)

Maximillian
(The Black Hole)

Mechagodzilla
(Godzilla vs the Bionic Monster)

Mega-Robots
(Robot Wars)

Mentor
(Star Virgin)

Metalogen Man
(The Monster and the Ape)

Miriam
(All You Zombies)
Mobus
(Johnny Wong: Hewo of the 21st Century)

Mogella
(Chikyu Boeigun)

Mouse Droids
(Star Wars I, IV, V, VI)

Muffet
(a Dagget) (Battlestar Galactica, Conquest of the Earth)

Newman
(And You Thought Your Parents Were Weird)

Nightdroids
(Pleasure Maze)

Nine-Eye
(From Time to Time)

Number 5 aka Johnny Five
(Short Circuit, Short Circuit 2)

Omega Doom
(Omega Doom)

Orus
(a clicker) (Creation of the Humanoids)

Otomo
(Robocop 3)

Patrol Droids
(Star Wars I, IV, V, VI)

Pax
(a clicker) (Creation of the Humanoids)

Pen Pals
(Escape from DS-3)

Percy
(The Ice Pirates)

Pioneer One
(I Love Maria)

Pioneer Two
(I Love Maria)

Pit Droids
(Star Wars I, IV, V, VI)

Pris
(a replicant) (Blade Runner)

Probe Droids/ Probots
(Star Wars I, IV, V, VI)

Protocol Droids
(Star Wars I, IV, V, VI)

Prowler
(Code of Silence)

Quantasaurus Rex
(Power Rangers Time Force – Quantum Ranger: Clash for Control)

R2-D2
(Star Wars I, IV, V, VI)

R-4
(The Lost Planet)

R-9
(The Lost Planet)

Rachael
(Blade Runner)

Rapist Robots
(Flesh Gordon)

R. Borgraf
(Robots)

R. Daneel Olivaw
(Robots)

Reformers
(Droid)

Refugee Robots
(A.I.: Artificial Intelligence)

Reiko
(I.K.U.)

Reilly
(Frankenstein Meets the Space Monster)

Replicants
(Blade Runner)

R. Giskard
(Robots)

R. Jane
(Robots)

Robby
(Forbidden Planet, The Invisible Boy)

Robot Q
(The Master Mystery)

Robovixens
(Batteries Included)

Rolo Droids
(Star Wars I, IV, V, VI)

Ro-Man
(Robot Monster)

Roms
(Omega Doom)

R.O.T.O.R.
(R.O.T.O.R.)

R. Sammy
(Robots)

RS1
(Tejing Xinrenlei 2)

Sammy, R.
(Robots)

Screamers
(Screamers)

Sith Probe Droid
(Star Wars I, IV, V, VI)

Sparks
(The Shape of Things to Come)

Spectre
(a Cylon) (Battlestar Galactica, Conquest of the Earth)

Synth
(Crash and Burn)

T-800 Terminator
(The Terminator, Terminator 2: Judgement Day)

T-1000 Terminator
(Terminator 2: Judgement Day)

Terminatrix
(Terminatrix)

Talkdroids
(Star Wars I, IV, V, VI)

Talos
(Jason and the Argonauts)

Tetra
(Jubunairu)

Thinko
(Sex Kittens Go To College)

TikTok's
(Return to Oz)

Tinpan
(Deadspace)

Tin Woodman
(The Wizard of Oz, The Wonderful Wizard of Oz)

Tobor
(Tobor the Great)

Tom Servo
(Mystery Science Theater 3000: The Movie)

Tracker
(Cybertracker)

Twiki
(Buck Rogers in the 25th Century)

Ulysses
(Making Mr Right)

Valcom-17485
(Heartbeeps)

Veronica
(Veronica 2030)

V'Ger
(Star Trek: The Motion Picture)

V.I.N.C.E.N.T.
(The Black Hole)

Volkites
(Undersea Kingdom)

Volto
(Robot Wrecks)

Voyou
(Armageddon:
The Final Challenge)

Wera
(Panenka)

Wesley Brenn
(The Lost Planet)

Yetis
(Downtime)

Zhora
(Blade Runner)

The idea of naming a kid after a robot may fill you with dread – it's illogical for a start, captain – but you can't rule it out as a possibility for the future. Especially when you consider the strange case of BRFXXCCXXMNPCKCCCC1 11Mmnprxv1mnckssqlbb11116. Have no fear, *SWAYCI*'s typing droid hasn't shortcircuited, nor has its spellchecker gone bonkers. According to the parents, this seemingly unpronounceable name is pronounced Albin. Apparently they fought hard against the Swedish authorities to give their son this futuristic name, but failed and copped for a £500 fine. The boy's mother is quoted as saying, "It is a pregnant, expressionistic typographic design that I see like an artistic new creation in the pathaphysical tradition that I join." Of course, it's so obvious! How could we have been so stupid?

Every year in Sweden, many parents' choice of name gets rejected. What a great idea. If the authorities think you're taking the piss, they fine you and stop you giving your kid a shit name. Shame they don't go a step further and pick a name themselves. Maybe some time in the future, eh?

Bizarrely, lots of other Swedish parents are almost as deranged as young Albin's. Names that have been approved by the powers that be include Summercloud, Jazz-Ture, Twilight, Månstråle (moonbeam), Fiddeli, Puma, Tiger and Texas. Names that didn't quite slip through include Lakrits (liquorice), Ikea Decibel, Blomsterblomma (flower flower), Måne (moon), Hosianna, Snövit (snow white), Filur (sly dog), Åskvigg and Bajen (the pooh). But what about the parents who wanted to call their baby Peter? Well, it would have been all right if the child had been a boy.

Left-field Swedes apart, as a continent, we're not far off a time when everyone will be a number. At the time of writing, national ID cards were being planned for the UK. Why not embrace the digital age now and give your kid a number for a name? You could be the one to start off a worldwide trend! Just don't forget the book that gave you the idea, OK?

In the cult 1960s TV show *The Prisoner*, Patrick McGoohan's Number Six claimed that he was a free man, not a number. He needn't have worried; in the future he could be both without being accused of being greedy.

Unlike letters, numbers have the great advantage that you can put them together in any sequence you like and they'll make as much or as little sense as any other sequence you've ever encountered. If all names in the future were numbers, there would be plenty of ways and means of creating a numeric name relevant to you, your partner or someone who inspired you. Any memorable date would be a good starting point. If you were particularly impressed by the first moon landing you could call your kid 210769, the date of Neil Armstrong's famous small step. A footy fan could name his kid after the last major trophy his team won, which would make *SWAYCI*'s author 150573. A darts fan could call his first-born 11 (eleven dart finish) or 170 (highest three-dart outshot). The list is endless and open to all sorts of naming creativity – far more, in fact, than any sequence of letters could possibly muster.

Numeric names are certainly worth considering. Millions of people are obsessed with their mobile phones, so why not name yourself after your mobile phone number? It would make things so much easier and prevent a lot of misdialling. You could take it a step further: if you are proud of where your child was born, use the local dialling code as the first few digits of its name. Similarly, if you want your child to join the police (hang on – why exactly?), you could simply call it 999. During those difficult, rebellious teenage years, it could claim it was named after the punk band.

Which leads us nicely to another fascinating area for conjecture. In the future, will kids' names be easily identifiable as male or female? If they were all given numbers, the answer would have to be a resounding "No."

In this day and age, when gender distinctions are blurring and becoming irrelevant, the natural next step is surely to go down the number road, or number line if you're a schoolteacher. Face it: by calling your child a number, you're going to shut up all the olds in your family, if nothing else.

Grandma X wanted Martha, whereas Grandma Y wanted Georgia. Tough luck, ladies. He's called 12345, and he's been named after the senses. No, he was actually named after the first five commandments. Or something. Who cares, anyway? With surnames like these, what right have the grandparents got to force their opinions on anybody?

In addition to obsessing over mobile phones, modern people like to spend time on the internet looking stuff up on search engines. In the future, a whole new breed of names will be chosen purely because they bring up exciting results on Google. What a great idea: instead of spending ages deliberating over the suitability of your kid's name, just whack in a few random letters and numbers and see what comes up. If you like what you see, use the name for your newborn. What could be easier?

Better still, name your nipper after a website you're particularly fond of, with the www. bit at the beginning and all the forward slashes in the right places. Whenever your kid is asked why the name, it can simply type it in the address bar and up pops the reason. To trump that idea, set up your own website, name your brat after it and update the site whenever the youngster achieves anything newsworthy. In today's climate of rewarding kids for the slightest thing, shitting its pants on a Tuesday should be reason enough to upload some new images on the home page.

As an alternative to such radical-sounding ideas, why not give all your kids a name followed by a version number? The first kid could be Adam Version 1.0 and his little brother Adam Version 2.0. If on the other hand you were feeling brave and the second kid looked just like the first, you could name him Adam Version 1.1. The system can't fail. It also gives you an easy way of remembering the relative ages of your children.

Don't like the idea? It's no more than a natural extension of what many Americans do already. Just look at the next US Open leader board and you'll see loads of Yanks with II or III or IV after their names, depending on whether they were called after their daddy, grandaddy or great-grandaddy.

Thing is, whether you're a name or a number you'll soon be on record for this, that and the other. It's unlikely that people will start naming their kids after numbers just yet, but in the digital age when you can do pretty much anything with a mobile phone or a PDA, the time when we'll all be numbers is probably a lot closer than we think. One of these days, robots will be running everything, and given the speed at which technology is moving they'll all be minute and incredibly clever. Who's going to be able to argue with a minute, incredibly clever, rock-hard android? Especially if it's been cloned several billion times. Which leads us perfectly to the subject of cloning humans and the implications for their names.

The vital question, of course, is should each clone be given the same name? They're all the same person, aren't they? Or should they all get different names, perhaps following the version system? Someone trying to keep tabs on them – a robot schoolteacher, say – would surely find it easier to refer to version numbers rather than have to spend all that valuable time thinking up and remembering names for them all.

Cloning is such a delicate subject these days, not least when it comes to the Raelian cult, which claims to have succeeded in cloning a human. Its leader, former French journalist and auto enthusiast Claude Vorilhon, who now styles himself Rael, claims to be a direct descendant of extraterrestrials who created human life on Earth through genetic engineering. A company founded by his followers announced that the first human clone had been born in 2002: a 7lb baby girl called Eve.

Understandably, Christian groups around the world were up in arms, especially about the choice of name. Come on guys, that's just so before Christ! It's true: the first cloned baby is named after the first woman in the Bible. How unoriginal. You'd have thought Claude Vorilhon, who came up with the oh-so-very-sci-fi name Rael (you can imagine him talking in a big, powerful, booming voice) could have done better than that.

Not surprisingly, much heated debate about whether cloning humans is a good idea and whether the Raelians actually did clone a person has been going on ever since.

So far, though, we've overlooked the biggest issue for everyone concerned: is having your own name a basic human right? Well, yes and no. Yes inasmuch as everyone deserves some form of identity; no when you consider that a simple name search on the Friends Reunited website will generally bring up 50-odd people who share the same name. Where's the dignity in that? Before we all descend into a mishmash of nuts and bolts, circuit boards, fake skin and programmed emotions, we need to get a grip on the situation and invent some new names, or at least give our kids a nudge in the right direction. Whatever you may think of Claude Vorilhon, at least he had the nous to change his name to something a bit space-age.

Given that the 26 letters in the alphabet offer a finite list of options, people in the future are going to have to consider naming their kids with a sequence of numbers. So let the grandkids decide. Since we'll all be waiting patiently in cryogenic suspension, we won't know any better for at least a few thousand years, by which time no one will give a shit about petty inconveniences like what we call each other. Although people may have discovered whether androids dream of electric sheep or not.

Sources
http://www.podster.pwp.blueyonder.co.uk

The great divide: Names that don't travel

8

A backpacker travelling around India was attempting to jump onto a very busy bus. He pleaded with the driver to let him on, but the harassed driver replied, "I'm sorry sir, I'm cram-jam full." The backpacker answered, "I don't care what your name is, mate, just let me on the bus."

Now that you've got this far, you're probably thinking, flippin' eck, are there any names left on this earth that I can choose for my kid that'll be any good? And you'd be right to think it. Never forget that the chances are that your kid will outlive you and will be stuck with its name unto death. A morbid thought, granted, but you'd be wise to bear it in mind from the moment you know there's a child on the way. As you've learnt by now, naming a child is a serious business.

Not many people think about this, but your child may not be born in the area or country that you come from, or it may want to move away when it grows up. (If this idea has occurred to you, congratulations, you're thinking the right way.) So what? Well, some names simply don't travel. This rule doesn't apply only to people's names. Take the Czechoslovakian town of Cheb. Or the German word for travelling, fahrt. Better still, the German word for father, *Vater*, pronounced farter. Straight away you'll be able to think of plenty of similar examples from foreign place names, terminology or brands.

If you thought the English were mean to Germans – even on a pseudo-acceptable "We won the war but we totally accept that your economy, standard of living and cars are far better than ours nowadays" level – that's nothing compared to the contempt in which they hold us. Germans hate the English so much that in Munich International Airport there's a thriving coffee shop that has as its façade a massive beige sign decorated with the word "bread" in 20 different languages – but not English. Not a big deal in the grand scheme of things, for sure; in general the Anglo-German hate thing is nothing more than a bit of Olaf these days. (Sorry, it's impossible to resist gags based around names not travelling.) Returning to the bread issue (notice how I cleverly change the focus of the paragraph), is it any wonder that the UK is such a mad place when people can't even agree on the name of a bread roll?

Check it out for yourself. Travel around the UK and you'll see that every fifteen miles there's a different name for a simple bread bun. Barms, muffins, cobs, stotties, bread cakes: they all mean much the same thing. But try and get someone to give you the definitive word on it and someone else will shout them down the moment the first crumb flies out of their mouth. If people can't agree on what to call a baked dough round, what chance do we have of finding a baby a name that someone somewhere doesn't find offensive, mispronounce or simply get wrong?

Consider Ford Prefect from Douglas Adams's *The Hitch Hiker's Guide to the Galaxy*. As an alien visiting earth, he researched common names but made the mistake of calling himself after a 1970s make of car, believing this would help him blend in. At least he got it right when he identified the towel as the most important part of a space traveller's luggage. To stick with matters Ford, *Viz* magazine once featured a letter purporting to come from an irate reader that wondered why the carmaker hadn't continued its policy of naming its new models after the titles of jazz mags. The reader claimed to have hoped that the Ford Escort and Ford Fiesta would be followed by the Ford Readers' Wives' Arseholes.

Although it could be argued that Ford Prefect made a reasonable fist of choosing a name that would slot into the social fabric of an unknown planet, his confidant Arthur Dent was blessed with a name that wouldn't even have crossed the English Channel. Arthur is perfectly acceptable, but dent is French for tooth. If he'd had to emigrate, or just popped over for a booze cruise, any French person who had cause to find out his surname would have barely been able to disguise their mirth. It's not as if the French need much excuse to take the piss out of the Brits.

Of course, we're not exactly immune to temptation ourselves. There must be millions of Germans named Klaus, but that doesn't stop them suffering when they come over here. Klaus the door behind you, will you? Don't stand so Klaus to me. Etc etc, to universal mirth. Travelling the other way, the nickname Dick, which is dying out fast in the UK for obvious reasons, means fat, thick or swollen in German. So is there an easy way to avoid giving your kid a name that doesn't travel? As ever, *SWAYCI* has the answer.

One cast-iron way of giving your child a name that will travel is to name it after something that can't *help* but travel. So here's a list of names that do travel. Rather quickly, in fact, since they're all names of hurricanes:

Alberto	Felix
Alex	Florence
Allison	Floyd
Ana	Frances
Arlene	Gabrielle
Arthur	Gaston
Barry	Gert
Bertha	Gordon
Beryl	Grace
Bill	Gustav
Bonnie	Hanna
Bret	Harvey
Chantal	Helene
Charley	Henri
Chris	Hermine
Cindy	Humberto
Claudette	Irene
Cristobal	Iris
Danielle	Isaac
Danny	Isabel
Dean	Isidore
Debby	Ivan
Dennis	Jeanne
Dolly	Jerry
Earl	Jose
Edouard	Josephine
Emily	Joyce
Erika	Juan
Erin	Karen
Ernesto	Karl
Fabian	Kate
Fay	Katrina

Keith
Kyle
Larry
Lenny
Leslie
Lili
Lisa
Lorenzo
Marco
Maria
Matthew
Michael
Michelle
Mindy
Nadine
Nana
Nate
Nicholas
Nicole
Noel
Odette
Olga
Omar
Oscar
Otto
Pablo
Paloma
Patty
Paula
Peter
Phelia
Philippe

Rafael
Rebekah
Rene
Richard
Rita
Rose
Sally
Sam
Sandy
Sebastien
Shary
Stan
Tammy
Tanya
Teddy
Teresa
Tomas
Tony
Valerie
Van
Vicky
Victor
Vince
Virginie
Walter
Wanda
Wendy
Wilfred
William
Wilma

The above list is currently in use by the World Meteorological Organization. Names are rotated on a six-year cycle, and "retired" if they become associated with a particularly devastating hurricane. The WMO's regional committee selects the names to replace those that are retired. Each year the names start with the "A" storm on that year's list, no matter how many names were used the previous year. Similar WMO regional committees are involved in selecting names for other parts of the world, but not all nations involved go along with these names. So some of these names will now be defunct.

To digress, one of the names above, Larry, is a common abbreviation of the name Laurence. Our crack team of researchers spoke to one Laurence whose mates called him Larry and then switched to La. When he passed his A levels and went off to university in Liverpool, all the locals thought his name was really Lad, as Scousers often say la for lad. If there's anywhere else in the world where a three-letter monosyllable routinely gets shortened, *SWAYCI* would like to hear about it.

In the Netherlands, Florence remains a perfectly proper name for girls, but whatever you do, don't abbreviate it to Flo as you might in England; it means flea in Dutch. The accepted abbreviation for Florence is Flor. (No wonder people tend to walk all over them. Ahem.)

Travelling eastwards, the Russians have many names that travel perfectly well: Aleksei, Aleksandr, Andrei, Denis and so forth. However, the country that gave us Lenin, Stalin and Gorbachev also possesses some absolute howlers. Take Sergei. When pronounced properly, it sounds just like Sir Guy. Imagine the hours of amusement that English-speaking countries around the world might get out of that:

"What's your name, comrade?"
"Sergei."
"Sir Guy?"
"Yeah."
"What did you get knighted for?"
"I didn't. That's my name."
"What, so, like, your parents decided to knight you? That's a bit posh, innit?"

Another common name in Russia is Igor. Can anyone think of it without imagining some lumbering oaf following Dr Frankenstein around and pandering to his every whim? Not much further down the list is Ivan; just add some possession or affliction to tap into a rich source of humour: Ivan Axe, Elbowinjury, Orriblewartonmyface *ad nauseam*. Russian nicknames are a good source of non-travelling mirth too. For example, Stanislav and Vyacheslav both become Slava, which may well be funny only if you were born and bred north of Birmingham. Vladimir, another common Russian name, is shortened to Vova, which admittedly isn't funny in the slightest unless you happened to be in the pub when one of *SWAYCI*'s mates insisted on calling this friendly Russian fella Vulva. (You had to be there at the time.)

And don't let's forget the corking Yuriy. Neither funny nor worthy of comment in its pure form, to be sure, but when its nickname of Yura rears its ugly head, well, there's a multitude of comic possibilities.

Russian girls, on the other hand, get off lightly; most of their names are demure, classy and regal-sounding. From Aleksandra, Alisa and Anzhelika through to Yuliya, Zinaida and the saucy Zoy, names for Russian females beat the ones available to the slightly more beardy sex hands down. We've established that to avoid piss-take, you should amongst other things ensure that the name you choose travels well. Failing that, make it your business to ensure your child grows up tough enough to handle any abuse that its name may attract.

Or you could fulfil both these obligations at a stroke by becoming a traveller. Descendants of nomadic traders and tinsmiths who emigrated to the United States 150 years ago, the Irish travellers have protected their culture by keeping the outside world at bay. The older folks among them still speak a Gaelic-derived language called Cant (careful how you pronounce it). Outsiders don't understand the travellers' language or their ways, but *SWAYCI* has uncovered some names for you in case you ever meet a traveller.

In Murphy village, Edgefield County, US (population roughly 3,000), there are but a dozen surnames, the most common being Carroll, Costello, Gorman, O'Hara and Sherlock. So many of the men have the same names that they go by nicknames such as Black Pete, White Man, Peekaboo and Mikey Boy.

Travellers throughout the world often use traditional forenames such as Samuel, William and Mary, but they are also fond of exotic names: Elijah, Goliath, Hezekiah, Nehemiah, Noah, Sampson, Shadrack, Amberline, Belcher, Dangerfield, Gilderoy, Liberty, Major, Nelson, Neptune, Silvanus and Vandlo for men, and Anselina, Athalia, Britannia, Cinderella, Clementina, Dotia, Gentilia, Sabina, Tryphena, Urania, Fairnette, Freedom, Mizelli, Ocean, Reservoir, Sinfai, Unity and Vancy for women. Surnames aren't quite so exotic, and are often shared by the Gorjer or non-traveller population. The best-known and most widespread include Ayres, Boswell, Buckland, Faa, Hearn, Heron, Lee, Lovell, Smith, Wood and Young.

Many travellers' surnames have fascinating origins. Travellers nearly always have a double nomenclature, with each tribe or family having a public name by which they are known to outsiders and a private name by which they are known amongst themselves. Public names usually sound quite English; private ones render these names into traveller equivalents.

Traveller names may be divided into two classes: names connected with trades and surnames or family names. In the first category, there are only two names that have been adopted by English travellers as proper names: Cooper and Smith. These names are expressed in English traveller dialect as Vardo-mescro and Petulengro. The first of these renderings is a bit far-fetched, as Vardo-mescro means cartwright. It would be nigh on impossible to render the word cooper into a traveller equivalent. A cooper is one who makes pails, tubs and barrels, and there are no traveller words for such vessels. Transylvanian travellers (no, not vampires) call a cooper a bedra-kero or pail-maker, but bedra is Hungarian, and English travellers might with equal propriety call a cooper a pail-engro. On the whole, the travellers did their best when they rendered cooper into their language as cartwright.

Petulengro, the other trade name, is borne by travellers who are known to the public as Smith. The name means horseshoe-fellow or tinker. Petali or petala signifies a horseshoe and is probably derived from modern Greek. The engro bit is either derived from or connected with the Sanskrit kara, to make, so Petulengro may be translated as horseshoe-maker. But bedel in Hebrew means tin, and as there isn't much difference between petul and bedel or between petul and petalon. Petulengro may be translated as tinker or tin-worker.

Tinkering is a principal pursuit of travellers. Whether you translate it as horseshoe-maker or tin-worker, Petulengro is as close to Smith as you'll get.

So much for trade names; now for family names. Many sound quite posh, and there's a good reason for this. When travellers first arrived in England, they sought the protection of powerful families who allowed them to pitch up on their heaths and woodlands. In time, the travellers came to adopt the names of their hosts. Here's a quick guide to some of the best-known English names for travellers, with their Romany equivalents:

Boswell

This name comes from the town of Bui. Bui or Bo is an old northern name signifying a colonist or settler, one who tills and builds. It was the name of many celebrated northern kempions (pioneering travellers), who won land and a home by hard blows. The last syllable comes from the French ville. Boswell, Boston and Busby all mean the same thing to the French, the Saxons and the Danish, and are half-brothers of Bovil (Beauville) and Belville, or fair town. The travellers confused bos with buss, meaning to kiss (easily done, to be fair), and so rendered the name Boswell as Chumomisto: Kisswell, or one who kisses well. Confusing? Yes, but choom in their language means to kiss, and misto means well.

Grey

This is the name of a family celebrated in English history. The travellers who adopted it bastardized the word gry, which means horse. They had no better choice, however, for in Romany and many other languages there is no word for grey. Maybe cos it's dull and they can't be arsed with it.

Hearne/Hearn

This is the name of a family that bears the heron for its crest. Either the name was derived from the crest, or the crest from the name. There are two traveller renderings of the word: Rossar-mescro or Ratzie-mescro and Balorengre. Rossar-mescro means duck-fellow (a bit harsh), the duck being substituted for the heron, for which Romany has no word. The meaning of Balorengre is hairy people (even harsher!) The translator may have confused Hearne with haaren, the Old English word for hairs.

Lee
The traveller name of this tribe is Purrum, sometimes pronounced Purrun. The meaning of Purrum is onion. "What connection is there between Lee and onion?" you may ask. Well, none, other than that they both go well with roast beef. You could argue that Lee sounds a bit like leek, giving us a vague vegetable connection.

Lovel/Lovell
This is the name of an old and powerful English family and means Leo's town, Lowe's town or Louis' town.

Marshall
The name Marshall comes either from the obvious source, a high military post, or from marches: not soldiers' rigid way of walking, but the borderlands where different countries meet. In the early Norman period, an Earl of Pembroke had this name. The travellers who took the name Marshall seem to have been convinced it was connected with marshes, as they rendered the name mokkado tan engre, or fellows of the wet or miry place.

Stanley
This is the name of another ancient English family and probably describes their original place of residence: a stony lea, which is also the meaning of the Gaelic Auchinlech, the place of abode of the Scottish Boswells. The name was adopted by an English traveller tribe. There are two Romany variations: Baryor/Baremescre (stone-folks or stonemasons) and Beshaley.

Beshaley is well worth a further look, and might help you impress someone down the pub one day. When Stanley was translated as Beshaley or Beshley, it was because someone mistook the stan bit for stand. Besh means to sit and ley or aley means down in traveller-speak. So why didn't they simply use the word for stand? Bizarrely, travellers have no such word in their language. But they had heard witnesses in courts of justice being told to stand down, so they reckoned standing down was the same as sitting down. In no travellers' dialect anywhere in the world is there a word for stand, though they all have a word for sit: besh. In every traveller encampment, Beshley or Beshaley is an invitation to sit down.

Right then, why don't you Beshley and consider the consequences of dreaming up a name that doesn't travel before you commit your kid to a life of immobility for fear of making itself a laughing stock the moment it crosses the road. That advice applies particularly if you're making something up or plumping for something foreign. Do your research! Find out where the name originates and have a sneaky look in the relevant English/*insert relevant foreign language here* dictionary in your local bookshop just in case it means something really stupid. The shop manager won't mind – they'll think you're clever. There's always a chance that changing a single letter in a name will make it mean something completely different and render it immediately acceptable in most countries around the world.

To sum up, if you don't know whether the name you're thinking of picking for your new kid means something dodgy in another language, don't use it. It's not worth the risk.

Sources

http://www.oceanrowing.com/hurricanes.htm
http://www.rickross.com/reference/irish_travelers/irish_travelers10.html
http://foclark.tripod.com/gypsy/surnames.htm
http://www.20000-names.com/gypsy_names.htm
http://www.globusz.com/ebooks/Romano/00000034.htm

Special thanks to Globusz Publishing for their permission to use material on travellers' names from their website www.globusz.com.

Kojak and other Telly names

9

Bond: You don't expect me to talk, do you?

Goldfinger: No, Mr Bond, I expect you to die!

In this chapter, *SWAYCI*'s crack team of researchers positioned strategically around the globe investigates some of the many memorable TV characters' names. Who knows, one of them may just come in handy for that troublesome moment when you have to think of a name for your sprog. We'll remind you about some unusual names that have appeared in a selection of long-running shows. We'll also slag animals off for no apparent reason.

From *Rainbow*'s wide-mouthed alien freak Zippy (because he's got a zip for a mouth, stupid) to the dull-sounding Miles Platting out of *EastEnders* (named after an area in north Manchester), scriptwriters and authors have to think up new names on a daily basis.

First, however, let us shatter your illusions. Sorry, it comes with the territory. Remember *Captain Pugwash*, the kids' cartoon? Didn't it have pirates in it called Seaman Stains and Master Bates and Roger the cabin boy? Sadly, no; it's an urban myth. Of course the cartoon existed; it was essential teatime viewing for a whole generation. But the characters were Captain Pugwash (obviously), Master Mate, Tom the cabin boy and bit-part pirates Barnabas and Willy. To help you show off in the pub, the ship was called the *Black Pig*. Oh yeah, and the rather jolly sea-shanty theme tune is the Trumpet Hornpipe, an anonymously composed traditional effort from Scotland, land of legends.

It's not exaggerating to say that many of us know more about certain TV characters than about our own friends and relatives. Similarly, many of us would be more inclined to name our children after telly characters than after famous poets, artists or writers. Regular viewers of, say, *Friends* (it's very popular among the *SWAYCI* team – yup, we're all in our 30s and don't get out much these days) know a fair bit about the background and life of the geeky Ross Geller. He has a doctorate in palaeontology, he worked at the New York Museum of Natural History before taking up a university teaching position, he's been married three times, he has two kids, he's Monica's brother, he's Jewish and so forth.

Many of us don't know nearly as much about our next-door neighbours or colleagues at work. Fictitious they may be, but we can't help getting to know (and care about) soap characters. Dirty Den, Sharon, Fred Elliott, Jim and Vera Duckworth, Nick Cotton, Mike Baldwin: they're all names that trip off the tongue. Admit it – you know all about them. You may not have thought about it, but we get to know TV characters in a different way from the way we get to know people in real life. What we find out about their lives, loves, jobs, habits and dreams is dictated by how much the shows' makers choose to show us. However much we'd like to, we can't ask our favourite characters how they feel about historical events or things that happened to them as children, and then build that information into our picture of them. What we know about them is carefully controlled to keep us intrigued and interested. Even the most basic information may be withheld from us so as to create watchable set-pieces, scenes and situations.

One common situation relying on incomplete information features in many long-running TV series: namely, leading characters whose names the audience never discovers, or who are often mentioned but never actually seen. Back in the swinging sixties, *Gilligan's Island*, a series about castaways marooned on an island in the South Pacific, concealed the full names of its main characters until late in the series. The series creator, the grandly named Sherwood Schwartz, apparently did this to make his castaways seem like archetypes rather than flesh-and-blood individuals. Pretentious rubbish or not, it must have appealed to the audience as it ran for three series, which made it quite a success in those days.

More recently, the multiple-award-winning British comedy *Only Fools and Horses* featured three characters whose full names were never revealed: the dim-witted roadsweeper Trigger, long-distance lorry driver Denzil and café owner Sid. In the hugely popular detective series *Inspector Morse*, the title character's first name, Endeavour, was kept secret until near the end of the 33-episode run.

Invisible characters are just as popular a device as incomplete names. Anyone who watched the 1980s classic *Minder*, starring George Cole as lovable rogue Arthur Daley and Dennis Waterman as Terry McCann, will remember that Her Indoors was Arthur's way of referring to the wife we never saw in the entire 15-year series. Mr Papadopoulis, Dot Cotton and Pauline Fowler's boss in *EastEnders*, didn't appear until the series had run for years, but was spoken about in passing almost every time there was a scene in the launderette. And Charlie from the glamorous 1970s cult show *Charlie's Angels* was heard over an office intercom in every episode, but never seen.

A certain Quentin Tarantino enjoys coming up with names for characters who don't appear in his movies, but he takes the idea a step further. He'll have a character mentioned in dialogue in one movie and bring them to life in the next, often in a lead role. Alabama Whitman, Mr White's ex-partner, makes no appearance in *Reservoir Dogs*, but features heavily in *True Romance*. We never see Bonnie in *Reservoir Dogs* or *True Romance*, but she plays a minor part in Pulp Fiction as Jimmy's wife. Marsellus Wallace (played by Ving Rhames – see the next chapter) doesn't appear in *Reservoir Dogs*, but is one of the main antagonists in Pulp Fiction. The list goes on, but *SWAYCI* will let you do your own research. We don't want to be branded as Tarantino bores. Tarantino *fans* if you will.

Anyway, whether you like Tarantino's movies or not (and how can you not?), the names he chooses are often memorable. On the other hand, some famous telly and film names are best avoided. Lassie, say, or Rin Tin Tin. Or Flipper, or Skippy. Let's be honest, who wants to be named after a dog? Or a dolphin? Or a kangaroo? Some names should never see the light of day on a human birth certificate.

No, if you're borrowing a name from the silver screen, make it a human one. Here for your convenience we've assembled a list of fantastic film characters' names (and credited the actors lucky enough to play them). If you want to name your child something slightly unusual without making it sound like a chav or a wannabe, you may find what you're looking for right here. We've even gone to the trouble of listing the name and year of the film in which a character appears so that you can check out a DVD before you commit yourself. Helpful or what?

You'll see that all the characters we list are pretty vivid personalities – maybe not role models, but people you can't help feeling strongly about. Even if none of the names strikes you as suitable for your new child, we hope they'll inspire you to think about your own favourite characters.

ACE VENTURA
(Jim Carrey): Ace Ventura: Pet Detective, 1994

ALABAMA WHITMAN
(Patricia Arquette): True Romance, 1993

AURORA GREENWAY
(Shirley MacLaine): Terms of Endearment, 1983

BEATRIX KIDDO AKA BLACK MAMBA
(Uma Thurman): Kill Bill, 2003

CLARICE STARLING
(Jodie Foster): Silence of the Lambs, 1991

DANIEL LARUSSO
(Ralph Macchio): Karate Kid, 1984

DARTH VADER
(David Prowse, voice James Earl Jones): Star Wars, 1977

DIL
(Jaye Davidson): The Crying Game, 1992

DOROTHY GALE
(Judy Garland): Wizard of Oz, 1939

ELLEN RIPLEY
(Sigourney Weaver): Alien, 1979

JOHN MATRIX
(Arnold Schwarzenegger): Commando, 1985

JOHN RAMBO
(Sylvester Stallone): First Blood, 1980

JUDAH BEN-HUR
(Charlton Heston): Ben-Hur, 1959

KEYSER SOZE
(Kevin Spacey): The Usual Suspects, 1995

HAN SOLO
(Harrison Ford): Star Wars, 1977

LULA PACE
(Laura Dern): Wild At Heart, 1990

MAD MAX ROCKATANSKY
(Mel Gibson): Mad Max, 1979

MATHILDA
(Natalie Portman): Leon, 1994

MONTY BREWSTER
(Richard Prior): Brewster's Millions, 1981

MORPHEUS
(Laurence Fishburne): The Matrix, 1999

RED
(Morgan Freeman): The Shawshank Redemption, 1994

RUFUS T. FIREFLY
(Groucho Marx): Duck Soup, 1933

SCARLET O'HARA
(Vivien Leigh): Gone With the Wind, 1939

SONJA
(Brigitte Nielsen): Red Sonja, 1990

STANLEY KOWALSKI
(Marlon Brando): A Streetcar Named Desire, 1951

THELMA & LOUISE
(Susan Sarandon, Geena Davis): Thelma & Louise, 1991

TONY MANERO
(John Travolta): Saturday Night Fever, 1977

TYLER DURDEN
(Brad Pitt): Fight Club, 1999

VERBAL KINT
(Kevin Spacey): The Usual Suspects, 1995.

Fans of *Casablanca* beware, though. Don't forget Bogart can easily be shortened to Bogey. Not even the cruellest parent would want a son or daughter to be named after a flickable nasal secretion.

Some people take the idea of borrowing names from films to extremes. One of *SWAYCI*'s crack researchers loved

Angel Heart so much that he named his four children after his favourite characters: Harold, Louis, Margaret and Epiphany. He's not totally off his head, he just got into a theme and stuck with it. Thankfully his wife's a fan too.

A friend of ours has three boys, David, Derek and Nigel. Nothing unusual there, you might think, but it just so happens they are named after the three members of the spoof rock band from the 1983 rockumentary *This Is Spinal Tap*. Speak to your mates: there'll be at least one who'll admit to having done something similar. For every ten kids with a normal-sounding name, one will be named after a character from their mum or dad's favourite film or TV show.

Most of the films we've looked at so far are American, and what we might call serious. If funny and British are more your style, you could do worse than use the Carry On films as inspiration. Take *Carry On Don't Lose Your Head*, based loosely on the story of the Scarlet Pimpernel and the French Revolution. The film opens at a Paris guillotine. "What's the tally for the day so far?" asks Citizen Camembert, the big cheese of the secret police, played by Kenneth Williams. "Twenty-six sets of aristos," answers his toadying assistant Bidet, played by Peter Butterworth. "Carry on chopping!" yells Camembert.

Sir Rodney Ffing (Sidney James) and his best mate Lord Darcy Pew (Jim Dale) are two workshy fops. To relieve the boredom, Sir Rodney becomes the Black Fingernail, a rescuer of French aristocrats from Madame La Guillotine who always leaves his calling card at the scene. The leader of the royalists, the Duc de Pommfrit (Charles Hawtrey), refuses to get off the execution cart to go to the guillotine because he's "Just on the last chapter of the latest Marquis de Sade." And so on. (Yes folks, we like Carry On as much as Tarantino.) The highlight comes when Camembert picks a duel with Sir Rodney. "As the injured party, I have the choice of swords or pistols," he proclaims. "Oh, we won't quarrel over that! You have the swords, I'll have the pistols," replies Sir Rodney, in a joke that predates *Raiders of the Lost Ark* by fourteen years.

Carry On Screaming, a Hammer horror pastiche, features some brilliant character names such as Constable Slobotham, Odd Bod, Junior and Detective Sergeant Bung. Have a look through the list below to see a few more. If nothing else, they'll give you a bit of a laugh.

ALBERT POOP-DECKER
(Bernard Cribbins): Carry On Jack

ALDERMAN PRATT
(Arnold Ridley): Carry On Girls

AUGUSTA PRODWORTHY
(June Whitfield): Carry On Girls

BERTRAM OLIPHANT WEST
(Jim Dale): Carry On Follow That Camel

BILIUS
(David Davenport): Carry On Cleo

BILL BOOSEY
(Sid James): Carry On Up the Jungle

BUNGHIT DIN
(Bernard Bresslaw): Carry On Up the Khyber

C. BOGGS
(Kenneth Williams): Carry On at Your Convenience

CITIZEN BIDET
(Peter Butterworth): Carry On Don't Lose Your Head

CITIZEN CAMEMBERT
(Kenneth Williams): Carry On Don't Lose Your Head

CONSTABLE CONSTABLE
(Kenneth Connor): Carry On Constable

DAPHNE HONEYBUTT
(Barbara Windsor): Carry On Spying

DETECTIVE SERGEANT BUNG
(Harry H. Corbett): Carry On Screaming

DR CARVER
(Kenneth Williams): Carry On Again Doctor

DR KILMORE
(Jim Dale): Carry On Doctor

DR NOOKEY
(Jim Dale): Carry On Again Doctor

DR TINKLE
(Kenneth Williams): Carry On Doctor

DUC DE POMFRIT
(Charles Hawtrey): Carry On Don't Lose Your Head

ESME CROWFOOT
(Joan Sims): Carry On Loving

GLADSTONE SCREWER
(Sid James): Carry On Again Doctor

GUNNER SHORTHOUSE
(Melvyn Hayes): Carry On England

HAROLD HUMP
(Henry McGee): Carry On Emmanuelle

IDA DOWNS
(Wendy Richards): Carry On Girls

JAMES BIND
(Charles Hawtrey): Carry On Spying

JUDGE BURKE
(Kenneth Williams): Carry On Cowboy

JOAN FUSSEY
(Joan Sims): Carry On Camping

KHASI OF KALABAR
(Kenneth Williams): Carry On Up the Khyber

MARCUS & SPENCIUS
(Gertan Klauber & Warren Mitchell): Carry On Cleo

MARSHALL P. KNUTT
(Jim Dale): Carry On Cowboy

MR DREERY
(Bill Maynard): Carry On Loving

MRS DANGLE
(Joan Sims): Carry On Emmanuelle

NURSE WILLING
(Elizabeth Knight): Carry On Again Doctor

PERCIVAL SNOOPER
(Kenneth Williams): Carry On Loving

PRIVATE WIDDLE
(Charles Hawtrey): Carry On Up the Khyber

PROFESSOR TINKLE
(Frankie Howerd): Carry On Up the Jungle

REVEREND FLASHER
(Sid James): Carry On Dick

SERGEANT JOCK STRAPP
(Jack Douglas): Carry On Dick

SERGEANT KNOCKER
(Phil Silvers): Carry On Follow That Camel

SIDNEY FIDDLER
(Sid James): Carry On Girls

SIR SIDNEY RUFF-DIAMOND
(Sid James): Carry On Up the Khyber

VIC FLANGE
(Sid James): Carry On Abroad

VIC SPANNER
(Kenneth Cope): Carry On at Your Convenience.

Anyway, enough of that Carry On. Some of *SWAYCI*'s older researchers would like to point out that if a particular name happens to feature prominently in a decent film and a good TV show around the same time, it will soon become a popular choice for naming newborn babies. This happens regardless of whether the TV show and film are related.

Consider the name Jason, bestowed upon innumerable boys from the mid-sixties to the early seventies. The film that started the ball rolling in 1963 was Don Chaffey's immense *Jason and the Argonauts*; the (completely unrelated) TV show to blame was the crime drama series Department S (first screened in 1968) and its even more camp spinoff *Jason King*, starring Peter Wyngarde. Just as interest in the film died down and Jason's popularity began to wane, it surged back with a vengeance thanks to a TV sleuth with big sideburns.

But TV exposure isn't a sure-fire recipe for a name's popularity. Some characters' names never catch on. A prime example is Homer from *The Simpsons*. Maybe it's because he's dim, fat and lazy that his name has yet to blaze a trail across the nation's primary-school classrooms. In years gone by, Homer was a perfectly acceptable name for a boy in the States, as Matt Groening's father could have attested. Until Mr Simpson came along and drank all the Duff, the name held positive associations, recalling the Greek epic poet who wrote the *Iliad* and the *Odyssey*.

That's enough on male names for now, don't you think? There's still a wealth of female characters' names to be trawled. We had a look at some of them earlier in the chapter, but there's a series of spy movies that's provided a rich vein of exotic girls' names for the past four decades or so. No prizes for guessing; it's time to give it up for the Bond girls. Nothing else sums up British culture, elegance and class like Pussy Galore, Honor Blackman's character in *Goldfinger*.

Bond is notorious for sleeping with nearly every woman he meets, apart of course from Miss Moneypenny. Men are old fashioned; they like to know their lovers' first names. She wouldn't tell, so he wouldn't sleep with her. Simple! Instead, 007 lavishes his attentions on a succession of succulently named females, Bibi Dahl, Elektra King, Fatima Blush, Holly Goodnight, Honey Ryder, Kissy Suzuki, Mary Goodnight, Molly Warmflash, Octopussy, Plenty O'Toole, Pussy Galore, Sylvia Trench, Vesper Lynn and Xenia Onatopp among them. Any of these names would immediately set your daughter apart from the crowd. She'd probably get beaten up a lot at school too.

Apart from considering the virtues or otherwise of the names themselves, you might want to think about the attitudes they represent. You do get some Bond fans (mainly men, amazingly enough) banging on about Bond girls being strong women in control of their lives. Oh yeah? Others would argue that they're just sex objects who exist solely to titillate men. Glamorous or not, Bond films are right up there with Benny Hill's TV shows in their crass and clichéd exploitation of women. Stick that in your pipe and smoke it, gentlemen!

Benny and Bond are both the stuff of 13-year-old boys' dreams. As far as we can make out, the only difference is the target viewer demographic, and there's not much in that, either. Benny Hill is for men who have lost all hope of seeing a naked girl in real life; James Bond is for men who still preserve the forlorn illusion that they might be able to go to bed with the women sitting next to them in the cinema. (And, we should say, it's also for the women sitting next to them, who like to think they have a chance of spending a night of passion with Mr Bond.)

Even so, the Bond movies do wield a certain amount of influence on the baby name charts. Whenever a new film comes out, the lead actor's name tends to surge in popularity. Look out for Sean (Connery), George (Lazenby), Roger (Moore), Timothy (Dalton) and Pierce (Brosnan) in the lists of years gone by. For a bonus point, does anyone know who played the very first James Bond? No, not Sean Connery in *Doctor No* in 1962, but Bob Holness, former *Blockbusters* presenter, on the radio in 1956. Would *SWAYCI* lie to you?

James Bond films are also a fine source of a different kind of name: the names of the super-villains that inhabit Bond's sophisticated yet dangerous world. How about naming your kid Auric (Goldfinger), Blofeld, Hugo Drax or Max Zorin? Better still, go for a name that struck terror into Bond fans and Peter Benchley readers alike: Jaws. Then again, that could be tempting fate: you wouldn't want your kid to grow up with dodgy teeth or to turn into a shark. Perhaps Oddjob would be a safer choice; you could get it to pop to the shop to buy your cigarettes and stuff.

It looks as though Bond wasn't the best place to look for girls' names. Just to even things up, let's have a last round-up of names from the telly and the movies that you might actually consider using for your daughter.

Callisto, from *Xena, Warrior Princess*, is a name from Greek myth meaning most beautiful. Jennifer (we're thinking of

Aniston, of course – everyone likes her) comes from the ancient Welsh Gwentwyfar, or Cornish Guinevere.

Nicole (from the Renault Clio series of ads, as in: "Nicole?" "Papa?") is, as you might guess, the feminine version of Nicholas. The original St Nicholas (forerunner of Santa) saved the daughters of a poor man from prostitution.

Roxanne (from the film based on *Cyrano de Bergerac* starring Daryl Hannah and Steve Martin) was the name of the wife of Alexander the Great (356–323 BC). Not to mention a hit single for the Police in 1979.

Tess (as in of the *D'Urbervilles*, played by Natassia Kinski, and Tess Daly, played by herself, as it were) means to reap. Tess was also the name of the supervising angel in *Touched by an Angel*.

Sources

http://tv.msn.com/tv/article.aspx?news=175617
http://www.tvshowboards.com/startrek/view.php?trd=041129232730
http://www.rotten.com/library/culture/james-bond/
http://www.snopes.com/radiotv/tv/nonames.asp
http://www.ofah.net/main.asp?page=433
http://www.tvacres.com/news_apr_2002_feature.htm
http://home.hiwaay.net/~warydbom/duesouth/thatname.htm
http://www.lowchensaustralia.com/names/famous.htm#4
http://rainbow.arch.scriptmania.com/rainbow_tv_episode.html
http://www.godamongdirectors.com/tarantino/faq/tarantinoverse.shtml
http://www.professorharbottle.co.uk/carryon.html

Silly-brity kids' names

A pregnant woman had a car accident and fell into a coma. She lay in a hospital bed for months. When she eventually woke up, she realized she was no longer pregnant and asked the doctor about her baby.

The doctor replied, "Congratulations. You had twins: a boy and a girl. Your brother came in and named them."

The woman asked, "What's the girl's name?"

"Denise."

"What about the boy's?"

"Denephew."

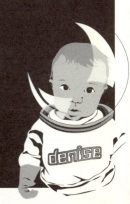

Fact: all babies look hideous when they're born. A bit like rats, really – at least until the umbilical cord has been cut. To be fair to the little blighters, they can look cute from the age of two to about 12, before they start going mad, getting spots and arguing with their parents all day. Once they're over that, they're adults and need to be taken seriously.

So why is it that celebrities don't think along these lines? A stupid name is a stupid name for life, not just for Christmas. It might seem like a laugh to choose a name while you're high on whatever the in substance is at the time, but it won't sound nearly as cute, trendy or thoughtful by the time your offspring hits puberty and starts hating you.

Put yourself in the bespoke box-fresh shoes of the average celebrity. Come on, at least try and imagine you've got no holes in your socks. Now imagine you've got millions of quid in your Swiss bank account, you own a house with more bedrooms, bathrooms and swimming pools than you'll ever need, and you can do just about anything you want, including giving your kid the daftest name under the sun. No, stop now. We're doing this the wrong way round. If you are a *real* celebrity, please heed this simple advice: when it comes to naming your child, imagine you're a pauper. Put those holes back in your socks. Money can't buy you love, nor can it buy you a great name for your baby.

There's a fair to middling chance Frank Zappa wasn't following our advice when he concocted the name Moon

Unit for his first child in 1967. Not content with having one of the world's maddest surnames, the late Mr Zappa felt it his duty to lumber his daughter with a name better suited to a spaceship. What made you do it, Frank? When Ford Prefect (see chapter 8) got it wrong, at least he had the excuse that he was from another planet: Betelgeuse, if memory serves. Maybe Zappa was on another planet too? It's only a theory...

Whatever you may think of Zappa's music or his choice of names, he made enough of an impact on the world to have a planet named after him, which is not something many of us can claim. Zappafrank was discovered by L. Brozek on 11 May 1980. For those of you with a telescope in your bedroom, it is thought to be between 4 and 8 miles in diameter. Its orbit is elliptical and approximately 4.08 years in duration, 193 million miles at perihelion and 282 million miles at aphelion. So now you know.

In fact, lots of people rate Zappa pretty highly. Kent Nagano, music director of the Opera de Lyon in Paris, said, "I was surprised that someone could be so multi-talented, such a good writer, and so articulate a composer. Moreover, he was a virtuoso technician on guitar and had an incredible sense of humour. He had all those skills and the ability to conceive, write, and orchestrate very complex orchestral scores." Matt Groening, creator of *The Simpsons*, hailed him as a genius: "Zappa didn't disguise his intelligence well enough. In addition to being a man of wide-ranging talent, one amazing thing that always struck me about Frank was his melodic dimension... Frank Zappa was my Elvis."

Sadly, Zappa died of prostate cancer in December 1993 at the age of 52. He is quoted as saying, "My job is extrapolating everything to its most absurd extreme." In naming his children Moon Unit, Dweezil, Ahmet Emuukha Rodan and Diva he certainly did that.

As it turns out, Moon Unit Zappa is a talented woman who has won the Aspen Comedy Award for Best Alternative Comic and written a novel and e-book entitled *America the Beautiful*. She lives in Los Angeles and single-handedly spawned the Valley Girl phenomenon when she sang backing vocals on the 1982 song of that name written and performed by her father.

A poll of 1,000 Brits between the ages of 18 and 65 posted on the internet in October 2004 gave Moon Unit the dubious honour of being voted the most bizarrely named celebrity offspring of all time. But competition was fierce. For a start, there was Fifi Trixibelle, the daughter of Bob Geldof and the late Paula Yates, who came second. And her sister Peaches (seventh), and half-sister Tiger Lily Heavenly Hirani (twelfth). Chris Martin and Gwyneth Paltrow's daughter Apple finished fourth, just behind Woody Allen and Mia Farrow's son Satchel. (It's never been proved that they use their son as a handy container for storing life's essentials, but it's a persistent mental picture nonetheless. Perhaps he grew up into a full set of ladies' and gents' matching luggage? Perhaps not.)

Next came Daisy Boo, the daughter of celebrity chef Jamie Oliver and wife Jools. Speculation as to whether the name meant the couple were fans of 1990s pop acts Daisy

Chainsaw and Betty Boo was unfounded. Daisy Boo was just ahead of Rumer, the daughter of Demi Moore and ex-husband Bruce Willis, in the top 20. We got a lot of fun out of her name at *SWAYCI* HQ. "Did you know Demi Moore's daughter is called Rumer?" someone would ask. "I heard that rumour." "I know, I started it." And so on. We didn't have much of a life in those days.

By the way, Moon Unit's brother Dweezil came thirteenth, and the elder Beckham boys, Brooklyn and Romeo, also made the top 20. Not even the royal family escaped the scorn of the great British public. Andrew and Fergie's daughter Princess Eugenie came fifteenth, just beating rhyming popstar couplets Rolan Bolan and Zowie Bowie.

Here's the full top 20, with the parents responsible in brackets:

1. MOON UNIT
(Frank and Gail Zappa)

2. FIFI TRIXIBELLE
(Paula Yates and Bob Geldof)

3. SATCHEL
(Mia Farrow and Woody Allen)

4. APPLE
(Gwyneth Paltrow and Chris Martin)

5. DAISY BOO
(Julia and Jamie Oliver)

6. RUMER
(Demi Moore and Bruce Willis)

7. PEACHES HONEYBLOSSOM
(Paula Yates and Bob Geldof)

8. RIVER
(Arlyn and John Phoenix)

9. ROCCO
(Madonna and Guy Ritchie)

10. NELL MARMALADE
(Helen Baxendale and David Eliot)

11. MADDOX
(adopted by Angelina Jolie)

12. HEAVENLY HIRANI TIGER LILY
(Paula Yates and Michael Hutchence)

13. DWEEZIL
(Frank and Gail Zappa)

14. BROOKLYN
(Victoria and David Beckham)

15. EUGENIE
(Sarah Ferguson and Prince Andrew)

16. ZOWIE
(Angie and David Bowie)

17. ROLAN
(Gloria Jones and Marc Bolan)

18. PHOENIX CHI
(Mel C and Jimmy Gulzar)

19. COCO
(Courtney Cox and David Arquette)

20. ROMEO
(Victoria and David Beckham)

At the time of writing, Apple was the fruit flavour of the month. Old Gwynnie (Paltrow) was delighted, to say the least. "The second that they put her on my chest, my life changed like that," she said, snapping her fingers. "My own ambition has sort of gone away, or at least, I have other priorities. Not only because of her birth, but I feel like I've accomplished so much when I was in my 20s, and I don't have that burning desire," she gushed. But let's be fair; the name wasn't her fault. "I didn't decide on the name, her daddy named her. I just liked the name. I got to give her her second name, Blythe, after my mother."

Why an apple? It's pure, apparently (try telling that to the greengrocer's at the end of our road) and comes from the earth. As do other fruits, of course. Claudia Schiffer named her daughter Clementine, as did former *Moonlighting* actress Cybill Shepherd. And let's not forget Peaches.

It makes you wonder why celebs seem to be compelled to choose off-the-wall names for their sprogs. One popular theory is that they're all intrinsically insecure about themselves, their talent and their fame. Bestowing a mad name on their kid is their way of attracting a bit more attention. Most celebs aren't famous for all that long, and they'll never reach the dizzy heights attained by the John Lennons, Marilyn Monroes and Elvis Presleys of this world. Or the next. Calling your child something peculiar doesn't make your fame last for ever, but it might drag it out for a few more years, even if it's only in idle conversation and dire TV nostalgia-fests.

Unfortunately for all us normal people, it's getting much easier to gain celebrity status these days, which means that the top 20 mentioned above will most likely swell to a top 50 or top 100 in the very near future. In those long-ago halcyon days when stars had to have some sort of talent, we might have forgiven them the odd foray into eccentric naming, yet John Lennon chose the eminently acceptable Julian and Sean as names for his sons, and Elvis picked the cute yet ageless Lisa Marie for his daughter. Poor old Marilyn Monroe never had any kids, but at least she made the effort to change her own name from plain old Norma Jean Mortenson.

Don't expect today's generation of charisma-free *Pop Idol* drop-outs, charmless *Big Brother* evictees or personality-bypass *Holiday Swap* contestants to apply any such decorum to their own naming choices. These people will do anything to be famous.

But we digress. Back to the established celebrities. How about Banjo and Audio Science? Fine names for a musical instrument and a degree subject, you might think, but they were in fact chosen as babies' names by actresses Rachel Griffiths and Shannyn Sossamon. And it gets worse. Start curling your toes now...

The two sons of moonwalking freak Michael Jackson are called Prince Michael I and Prince Michael II (nicknamed Blanket). How modest is that? In keeping with the royal theme, Jermaine Jackson has a child named Jermajesty. It beggars belief, but it's true. Fear not, for surely one day all celebrities will disappear up their own arses. Until then, though, let's stick with the naming and shaming.

In 2004, Jason Lee (the actor, not the curiously coiffed footballer) and his fiancée Beth Riesgraf named their son Pilot Inspektor. They offered no explanation for this eccentric choice, leaving everyone to wonder if someone in the family worked for the gas board.

For personalities of a certain age, the hippie-dippy factor may play a part. Cher had Chastity – oh, how ironic – with Sonny, and Elijah Blue with Greg Allman. David Bowie's son Zowie predictably tired of his name and started calling himself Duncan, then Joe. Grace Slick and Paul Kantner of prog-rock band Jefferson Airplane took the communion wafer when they let it slip that they were planning to call their daughter god (yes folks, with a small g), but settled in the end for China (they at least had the good grace to use a capital C) after running into resistance from bureaucrats when it came to filling in the birth certificate.

Time and again, pop stars, rock stars and thesps are guilty of naming crimes. Actress Bijou Phillips is the daughter of the late John Phillips of the Mamas and the Papas. Spare a thought for US actor Rob Morrow's daughter, Tu. Think about it for a little while, then think yourself lucky. Sylvester Stallone's five children share the Italian Stallion's alliterative affliction. He had Sage and Seargeoh with his first wife and Sophia, Sistine and Scarlet with current wife Jennifer Flavin. If that seems a bit vain, it's nothing compared to ex-boxer George Foreman, who named his sons George Jr, George III, George IV, George V and George VI. Girls presented a bit more of a problem, but he couldn't resist calling one of his five daughters Georgetta. Apparently he likes to joke that he can't remember his sons' names. Hilarious. Not that any of the *SWAYCI* team would keep a straight face if he told that particular gag within punching distance.

The late Emlyn Hughes, former captain of Liverpool and England football teams, called his son Emlyn and his daughter Emma Lynn. Really. For all his tenacious tackling and leadership qualities, here was someone who clearly wanted his name to live on.

But let's not spend all our time picking fault. As if. A few names that have sprung up in recent years are worth considering. We might even say they're cool. John Travolta and Kelly Preston's son is called Jett. Erykah Badu and Andre Benjamin (aka Andre 3000) named their kid Seven Sirius. Toni Braxton's son is Denim; whether she follows this up with Corduroy, Cotton or Polyester is up to her. Elle MacPherson's son is Aurelius Cy (taken from Ancient Rome, you know). Rob Thomas, co-writer of *Dawson's Creek*, has a daughter called Maison, French for house (obviously he didn't heed our advice about names that travel).

Ving Rhames (real name Irving), who played gangster Marsellus Wallace in *Pulp Fiction*, has kids called Reignbeau and Freedom. Who are we to question his choices, we add (just in case he decides to get medieval on our hillbilly asses)? Tea Leoni and David Duchovny named their baby Kyd. At least it's easy to remember: "Hey, Kyd!" Rock guitarist John Cougar Mellencamp's son is called Speck Wildhorse. Again, you're not gonna forget a name like that in a hurry. P. Diddy's daughter is called Lashanda Pawnesha Diddy – a chav name if ever there was one (see next chapter). Fellow US musician Tori Amos's daughter copped for the unusual Faerie.

If you've read this far you'll be thinking that all *SWAYCI* does is mock and criticize. And you'd be right. But we are capable of treating our best-loved celebrities with sensitivity. Allow us to justify and condone a couple of choices made by a famous movie actress and her partner in 2004. Congratulations, Mr and Mrs Julia Roberts, on the birth of your twins, Hazel and Phinnaeus. But our joy over your blessed event is tempered by a question. Why Phinnaeus? We know we don't live in a Janet, John and Mary era any more, and the traditional honour-thy-ancestors consensus of previous generations has collapsed under the weight of all those Britneys and Justins. But Phinnaeus?

Hazel is retro – the free world stopped giving birth to Hazels around the time it stopped having Berthas, Gladyses and Mildreds – but acceptable. Once the Pill became readily available and chemists started opening longer hours to suit men in search of condoms, choosing babies' names became more of an art form and less of a chore. But Phinnaeus went out with the ark – almost literally, as it dates back to the Old Testament, where it kept company with the likes of Methuselah and Obadiah. Still, give the Roberts some credit. They weren't reinventing the wheel, nor were they making names up for the hell of it. At least their twins will grow up in the knowledge that their names weren't hand-crafted for the occasion by their famous parents.

Psychologist Cleveland Kent Evans, who studies names and their social effects (as well he might), says the fancy-name trend among celebrities is a kind of self-reinforcing phenomenon. "I don't think of these names as coming just from celebrities so much as coming from creative celebrities, or at least those that want to be thought of as creative," he says. It's musicians and actresses and artists, not politicians and athletes, who choose wacky names for their kids. His observation certainly rings true in the US. Senator John Edwards and his wife Elizabeth called their youngest children by the pleasantly pedestrian names of Jack and Emma Claire. Similarly, ice-hockey great Wayne Gretzky and his actress wife Janet Jones contented themselves with Ty, Trevor, Tristan and Paulina.

Brown University professor Lewis P. Lipsitt, an expert in human development, says children's names can have positive and negative social consequences, but tend to be less important to their well-being than other factors such as their relationship with their parents. He speculates that unusual names are a way to give a celebrity's child: "A chance to be distinctive in [their] own right instead of just being known as [Celebrity X's] child."

So let's be fair to celebs. They may be acting out of the best motives after all. In any case, there are hard-to-digest names aplenty out here in the non-celebrity world too. It wasn't a famous person who had his name legally changed to Trout Fishing in America. That's right: *Mr* Trout Fishing in America, to you.

Sources
http://www.zappa.com/cheezoid/
http://cfa-www.harvard.edu/cfa/ps/mpc.html
http://www.funnynames.com/
http://www.amiright.com/names/siblings/index.shtml
http://www.funtrivia.com/dir/4806.htm

Chardonnay, madam? The world of the chav

Child: Mummy, why are your hands so soft?

Mother: Because I'm thirteen

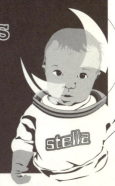

To get into character to write this chapter, *SWAYCI* has cracked open a four-pack of Stella, sparked up a Lambert & Butler, switched on *Trisha*, kicked the Staffordshire bull terrier back into the kitchen and donned the following items of clothing:

A pair of white Reebok classics (the Rockports got a bit muddy after last night's police chase through a field after we abandoned the stolen car)

A pair of white sport socks

A pair of tracksuit bottoms (only Nike or Adidas, mind) tucked into aforementioned socks

Lacoste polo shirt (the horizontally striped Fred Perry got stolen off the washing line)

Tracksuit top (Nike or Adidas again)

Chunky gold chain around neck, sovereign rings on fingers, gold earrings, bleached-blond hair, Burberry cap, and optional bum-fluff moustache.

And that's just the girls.

Thing is, as you've just seen, chavs have such a tribal dress code that you can spot one yards away. Not that you'll often see a chav on their own; they tend to appear in packs, like dogs. Everything they wear has to be branded, too, with brands of choice being Adidas, Nike,

Stone Island, Rockport, Lacoste, Nickelson, Hackett, McKenzie and Burberry. Their whole dress sense is entirely determined by what name's on the label, regardless of how ridiculous it looks, whether it fits and whether it clashes wildly with whatever else they've got on.

Worse, though, everything they do has to be seen as hard or cool in some way whenever a fellow chav is watching. This tends to encourage dirty deeds like mindless violence, vandalism, casual drug abuse or the wearing of chunky gold jewellery with intent. Thankfully, chavs aren't much like normal folk, but they do share something with us. They all have names.

It's only right and proper to start with the name chav itself. There are various theories about where it comes from, one of the most common being that it's merely an abbreviation of Cheltenham average, a street rat common in the Essex area. A writer on the *Independent* suggested that it derives from Chatham, in Kent. The term can be applied loosely to any culture with a nasty thieving element, but it may originate from gypsies, many of whom have lived in the area for generations. The Romany word for a child, chavi, was first recorded in the middle of the nineteenth century. *SWAYCI* has it on good authority that it was used to denote an adult man at that time too, but it hasn't often been recorded in print since – until now, of course.

From a linguistic perspective, the most fascinating aspect of chavs is the wide variety of local names they attract. Scots call them neds. Depending on who you believe, this is either an acronym for non-educated delinquents or a variant on teddy boys (named after their preference for an Edwardian style of dress). As we all know, especially those of us who used to watch *Brookside*, Scousers use the term scallies. In London, the prevailing name is kev, presumably from Kevin, an idiotic teenage character created by Harry Enfield and a common name among chav types.

Other terms recorded from various parts of the country are janners (Plymouth) and smicks, spides, moakes and steeks (all from Belfast; good work, Belfast! – some top names there). Bazzas works on the same principle as kev, baz being short for Barry, another popular chav name. Then there's charvers (from north-east England) and kappa slappers (promiscuous girls who wear Kappa-brand tracksuits). In the US, their closest equivalents are known as white trash or trailer (park) trash, alluding to their pasty complexions and choice of low-quality, low-maintenance living space.

If you're still confused as to the true definition of chav, for it goes far beyond their poorly developed taste in clothing (try and picture Welsh rap band Goldie Lookin Chain for reference), let our researchers offer a few of their own insights into the matter.

Though they love movies, especially on pirate DVD – which really gets their tongues wagging and saliva dripping – chavs aren't fussed about special features, actor interviews, director's cuts and the like. All they're concerned about is the amount, nature and extremity of violence, swearing and nudity. Discussions heard in chav circles are not about how wonderful a certain actor is at portraying particular characters, but rather about how hard he is and would he be able to knack/tub/burst/leather/hammer/tatter/batter Vin Diesel, Arnie, Bruce Willis, Sylvester Stallone, Chuck Norris, Bruce Lee and so on. Unsurprisingly, many chav children (chavdren) cop for the above names. Nor would chavs comment on a leading lady's conviction or empathy; their only interest is whether she has big tits or shows her fanny. There's a fair chance chavs may have heard of Spielberg and Lucas, but they probably think they're the same person.

Chav taste in films is pretty predictable: gangster movies, martial arts movies, action movies, teenage slasher fests and any combos thereof (gangster/action movies, martial arts/horror movies, horror/action movies, action/slasher movies. . . you get the idea). Gangster movies are a particular favourite, which makes the likes of *Goodfellas*, *Casino* and *The Untouchables* rich sources of chav names. The characters in these films, with their horrifically anti-social traits, are role models for chavs. Look out for teenage chavs called Henry, Jimmy and Tommy – the most violent, evil and malevolent characters from *Goodfellas*, all three based on real people who committed various heinous crimes. That's chavs for you – they've got a whole different value system to everyone else.

Being obsessed with anything villainous and violent, they often get into a few scrapes. To make their names sound appropriately menacing, they often add some kind of description or title, in the style of real-life gangsters like Jack "the Hat" McVitie and "Mad" Frankie Fraser. You don't have to meet them to know they're gangsters. They just sound like gangsters, More often than not, such names are secretly thought up by the gangsters (or wannabe gangsters) themselves.

John L. Smith's excellent novel *Of Rats and Men* features some fantastic gangster names that most chavs would give their left Rockport for: Tony "the Ant" Spilotro, Sam Giancana, Tony Accardo and Joey "the Clown" Lombardo. Apart from their ingenuity with alibis, lies and excuses, chavs aren't known for their imagination, so don't be surprised if you read about the likes of "Rockport" Johnny Smith, Jimmy "the Burberry" Brown or "Fat" Kev Jones in the name and shame page of your local newspaper.

Although chavs are fond of many names, especially if they're brand names, what struck the *SWAYCI* team, when we dared hang around long enough, was that many chavs seem to put more effort into naming their pets than they do their children. (This goes for caring for them too. A chav's last 50p is more likely to be spent on dogfood than food for their family.) Chavs love naming their dogs after boxers, cats after drugs and goldfish after R 'n' B artists. For every chav family, there's a vicious dog called Tyson or Bruno, an edgy cat called Charlie or Spliff and an oppressed goldfish called R. Kelly or Jamelia.

If only chavs applied the same imagination to their own names. Any name with one syllable gets an extra vowel sound shoved on the end; conversely, any name that's two syllables or longer is shortened to one syllable. Elegant names are rendered charmless by the sheer indolence of chav speech: Natasha becomes Tash, Victoria Tor and

Elizabeth Bet (not just a name but a popular pastime chez chavs). All this is indicative of their many other undesirable habits, which can be summed up as lazy, negative and violent.

The popular Channel 4 TV series *Max and Paddy*, featuring two hapless doormen roaming the country in a van, will no doubt prompt an upsurge in chavs of those names. Whenever chavs identify traits they like in TV characters, especially lovable rogues, they soon nick their names and use them for the next generation of undesirables.

Chavs know the price of everything – especially when it comes to sports brands, cars and plasma tellies – and the value of nothing. What counts as an achievement for a chav is to appear on a show like *Trisha* (a common chav name; give the girl some respect, man), instead of just sitting at home watching it in the company of a supersize McDonalds. (Ron is a common chav name too, though a chav would never make the link. Let's hear it for Ronald!)

Chavs are completely without morals, having never been taught about right and wrong by their inattentive, uncaring and frequently absent parents. Maybe this explains why many of them reject their real names for snappy nicknames. Face it, if your mum or dad constantly roared your name followed by a threat if you didn't do or stop doing something, you'd soon get sick of the sound of it. One thing chavs never tire of, however, is possessions with a high perceived value, especially chunky clunky gold jewellery or titchy tiny mobile phones. A chav is part magpie, lover of all things shiny – or bling, as vacuous, illiterate street slang would say.

Whatever their ethnic background, chavs have a built-in affinity to hip-hop and R 'n' B, even if they are inherently racist. They see their life as glamorous and cool. For the most part, they are extremely stupid. However, some possess a form of low cunning that can be misinterpreted as intelligence. Chavs have no desire to better themselves through honest means nor to learn anything outside car modification, what's new on the McDonald's menu and how much the latest Burberry scarf costs.

All chavs think that they are as hard as nails, hence their love of tough movies. But if you want to know what they are really like, the TV series *Shameless* and *The Royle Family* offer fine examples of the way chav families conduct themselves. Or look at the Bacon family in Viz, or Matt Lucas's grotesque teenage mother in Little Britain. Chavs are incredibly fertile beasts, and highly successful breeders. Where they come unstuck is in looking after the offspring produced by their drunken underage fumbles. More often that not their unfortunate child will grow up to be another chav, having received no more guidance on life than its parents did.

Chavs spend more money on their car exhausts, wheel trims and stereo systems than they do on their children. In fact, the only major financial commitment to a newborn chav is a pair of earrings and the cost of the piercing before it cuts its first tooth. But though they love cars, they have a funny way of showing it. Rather than buy a decent motor to start with, chavs spend all their unemployment benefit, sickness pay and tax-free labouring cash on upgrading a ten-year-old car with at least 180,000 miles on the clock. The end product will inevitably be a luminous, noisy, large-exhausted monstrosity (a chaviot, in fact) with at least one fatal or near-fatal collision to its name. The magazine *Max Power* has a lot to answer for.

Chavs like to hang around the takeaway of an evening, as the shopping centre has usually closed for the night by then. We can exclusively reveal that this habit exerts a formative influence over the names they choose for their kids when they inevitably give birth in their teenage years. From the perennially popular Bombay (usually a middle name rather than a first name) all the way to Tikka Masala, takeaway menus provide a ready source of names for chav babies, some of which are even home delivery. See what we did there? The names Marina, Nacho, Rogan, Romana and Toscana are equally easy to trace back to a bit of laminated plastic stuck in a window.

In much the same way, the anti-social habits of under-age drinking, smoking, talking bollocks and starting fights in queues all give rise to common chav names. One teenage chav had the following conversation with his probation officer:

"So, you've got a baby. Stella: what a beautiful name. Have you changed your ways and started studying Ancient Roman culture, language and mythology?" asked the probation officer.

"You what?"

"Well, Stella means star in Latin."

"Really? I just named her after the lager I was drinking when she was born."

Not just booze but fags as well have been adopted as children's names. One girl who recently gave birth to twin boys named them Lambert and Butler. Her bezzie mate followed suit and called her sons Benson and Hedges. Another popular chav name nowadays is Carly, after Carling. Another chav couple (a rare thing; parents are usually estranged within weeks) handed their kid the name Billy. Surely that's not too bad? It is when you know the reason: both parents are regular users of speed, otherwise known as Billy Whizz.

To be fair, chav mothers probably can't spare the time to put much effort into naming their kids. The *Daily Mail* summed up the style of the female chav (or chavette) admirably. As well as favouring flashy gold jewellery (hooped earrings, thick neck chains, sovereign rings and heavy bangles, all of which come under the catch-all term bling), wearing prison-white trainers (they're so pristine they look new), and sporting clothes with conspicuous logos and baseball caps, preferably by Burberry, all chav women "Pull their shoddily dyed hair back in that ultra-tight bun known as a 'council-house facelift,' wear skirts too short for their mottled blue thighs, and expose too much of their distressingly flabby midriffs." Is it any wonder they don't spend long choosing their kids' names when they're so busy making themselves beautiful?

This upsurge of popular distaste towards chavs may be evidence of a cultural shift back to a class-conscious society – at least, that's what they worry about in liberal circles – but that's not for us to judge. What we're concerned with is the ins and outs of chav naming, right?

Most common chav names – Baz, Daz, Gaz, Shaz, Steve and Trace – share a common thread. Chavs aren't clever enough to get their heads around long names, and even if they could, they'd be far too lazy to say them. Their leaders, who distinguish themselves by being able to utter names as long as two syllables, put a cunning twist on these abbreviated names by adding an a, o or y on the end. What they are too stupid to realize is that this makes the nicknames just as long as the original names from which they were derived. But don't say that to their face or you'll get a battering. Or at least a threat of one.

Another defining characteristic of chav culture is choosing a name that grates on everyone else. This technique is most effective when you've got a strong regional accent. If you're a scouser, say, simply choose a name with a few Ts in it. Every time you say it, you'll shower everyone in a five-metre radius with spit. Straight away your kid's name will assume chavdom, simply because of the way it's pronounced.

Anyone trying to avoid inadvertently choosing a chav name for their baby needs to know that chav names go in and out of fashion. Once your child is dragged down into chavdom, it's hard to rise back out of it; before you know it, your lovely little Lesley-Ann with the pink frock is suddenly simply Lez, and wearing the highest of heels and the miniest of skirts. But one failsafe way of identifying a chav kid is to find out who the media darlings were when it was born. *SWAYCI* confidently predicts a steady rise in Jordans, Peters, Jermaines, Anthonys and Declans over the next couple of years.

As decent human beings, the names we give our children should reflect something deeper than devotion to a football team, enthusiasm for a TV show or loyalty to a label. That's the stuff of chavs. Let's name our children after people who embody the virtues to which we would have them aspire. We should bless our kids with the names of holy women and men – or at least names that won't go out of fashion the moment Top Shop brings out its autumn collection – and leave the names of footballers for our pets.

One guaranteed way of avoiding a chav name is to pick something that a chav would never think of using. How? Simple. Pick a character from Shakespeare. The only Shakespeare a chav will have been into is the pub down the road. Here, with our thanks to babynames.org.uk, is a selection of some of the names used in Shakespearean plays; we've even included the posh pronunciation bit afterwards, just in case this book falls into the hands of a chav.

ADRIANA
(ad-ri-â'-nå)

AEGEON
(ê'-ge-on)

AEMILIA
(ê-mil'-i-å)

ALCIBIADES
(al-si-bî'-å-dêz)

ALIENA
(â-li-ê'-nå)

ANDROMACHE
(an-drom'-akê)

ANGELO
(an'-je-lô)

ANTENOR
(an -te'-nër)

ANTIOCH
(an'-ti-ok)

ANTIOCHUS
(an-tî'-o-kus)

ANTIPHOLUS
(an-tif'-o-lus)

ANTONIO
(an-tô'-ni-ô)

APEMANTUS
(ap-e-man'-tus)

APOLLO
(å-pol'-ô)

ARIEL
(â'ri-el)

ARRAGON
(ar'-å-gon)

BANQUO
(ban'-kwô)

BAPTISTA
(bap-tis'-tå)

BASSANIO
(bas-sa'-ni-ô)

BEATRICE
(bê'å-tris)

BELLARIO
(bel-lâ'-ri-ô)

BELLARIUS
(bel-lâ'-ri-us)

BENEDICK
(ben'-e-dik)

BENVOLIO
(ben-vô'-li-ô)

BERTRAM
(bër'-tram)

BIANCA
(bê-an'-kå)

So, what are you calling it? > 178

BORACHIO
(bô-rach'-i-ô)

BRABANTIO
(brå-ban'chô)

BURGUNDY
(bür'-gun-di)

CALIBAN
(kal'-i-ban)

CALCHAS
(kal' -kas)

CAMILLO
(kå-mil'-ô)

CAPULET
(kap'-û-let)

CASSIO
(kas'-i-ô)

CELIA
(sê'-li-å)

CENTAUR
(sen'-tawr)

CERIMON
(sê'-ri-mon)

CESARIO
(se-sâ'-ri-ô)

CLAUDIO
(klaw'-di-ô)

CLAUDIUS
(klaw'-di-us)

CORDELIA
(kawr-dê'-li-å)

CORNWALL
(kawrn'-wawl)

CYMBELINE
(sim'-be-lên)

DEMETRIUS
(de-mê'-tri-us)

DESDEMONA
(des-de-mô-nå)

DIANA
(dî-an'-å)

DIONYZA
(dî-ô-nî'-zå)

DONALBAIN
(don'-al-ban)

DORICLES
(dor'-i-klêz)

DROMIO
(drô'-mi-ô)

DUNCAN
(dung'-kån)

EMILIA
(ê-mil'-i-å)

EPHESUS
(ef'e-sus)

ESCALUS
(es'-kå-lus)

FERDINAND
(fër'-di-nand)

FLAMINIUS
(flå-min'-i-us)

FLAVIUS
(flâ'-vi-us)

FLEANCE
(flê'-ans)

FLORIZEL
(flor'-i-zel)

FORTINBRAS
(fôr'-tin-brås)

GANYMEDE
(gan'-i-mêd)

GIULIO
(jû'-li-ô)

GONERIL
(gon'-e-ril)

GONZALO
(gon-zah'-lô)

HELENA
(hel'-e-nå)

HELICANUS
(hel-i-kâ'nus)

HERCULES
(hër'kû-lêz)

HERMIA
(hër'mi-å)

HERMIONE
(hër-mî'-o-nê)

HORATIO
(hô-râ'-shi-ô)

HORTENSIO
(hor-ten'-si-ô)

IACHIMO
(yak'-i-mô)

IAGO
(ê-ah-gô)

ILLYRIA
(il-lir'-i-å)

IMOGEN
(im'-o-jen)

JESSICA
(jes'-i-kå)

JULIET
(ju'li-et)

LAERTES
(lâ-ër'-têz)

LAFEU
(lah-fu')

LEAR
(lêr)

LEODOVICO
(lê-ô-dô'-vi-kô)

LEONATO
(lê-ô-nâ'-tô)

LEONTES
(lê-on-têz)

LUCIANA
(lû-shi-â'nå)

LUCIO
(lû'-shi-ô)

LUCIUS
(lû'-shi-us)

LUCULLUS
(lû-kul'-us)

LYSANDER
(lî-san'-dër)

LYSIMACHUS
(lî-sim'-å-kus)

MACBETH
(mak-beth')

MAGDALEN
(mag'-då-len)

MALCOLM
(mal'-kum)

MALVOLIO
(mal-vô'li-ô)

MANTUA
(man-'tû-å)

MARIANA
(mah-ri-â'-na)

MENAPHON
(men'-å-fon)

MERCUTIO
(mer-kû'-shi-ô)

MESSINA
(mes-sê'-nah)

MILAN
(mil'-ån)

MIRANDA
(mî-ran'-då)

MONTAGU
(mon'-tå-gû)

MONTANO
(mon-tah'-nô)

OBERON
(ob'-ër-on)

OLIVIA
(ô-liv'-i-å)

OPHELIA
(ô-fêl'-i-å or o-fêl'-yå)

ORLANDO
(awr-lan'-dô)

ORSINO
(awr-sê'-nô)

OTHELLO
(ô-thel'-ô)

PAROLLES
(pa-rol'-êz)

PAULINA
(paw-lî'-nå)

PENTAPOLIS
(pen-tap'-o-lis)

PERDITA
(për'-di-tå)

PERICLES
(per'-i-klêz)

PETRUCHIO
(pe-trû'-chi-ô)

PHOENIX
(fê'-niks)

PISANIO
(pê-sah'-ni-ô)

POLIXINES
(pô-liks'-e-nêz)

POLONIUS
(pô-lô'-ni-us)

PORTIA
(pôr'-shi-å)

PROTEUS
(prô'-te-us or prô'-tûs)

REGAN
(rê'-gån)

RODERIGO
(rô-der'-i-gô)

ROMANO
(rô-mah'-nô)

ROMEO
(rô'-me-ô)

ROSALIND
(roz'-å-lind)

ROSALINE
(roz'-å-lin)

So, what are you calling it?

Rousillon
(ru-sê-lyawng')

Sebastian
(se-bas'-ti-ån)

Sempronius
(sem-prô'-ni-us)

Simonides
(si-mon'-i-dêz)

Solinus
(sô-lî'-nus)

Sycorax
(sî'-ko-raks)

Syracuse
(sir-å-kus)

Thaisa
(tha-is'-å)

Thaliard
(thâ'-li-ård)

Thurio
(thû'-ri-ô)

Timon
(tî'-mon)

Titania
(tî-tan'-i-å)

Tybalt
(tib'-ålt)

Ursula
(ur'-sû-lå)

Venetian
(ve-nê'-shån)

Venice
(ven'-is)

Ventidius
(ven-tid'-i-us)

Verona
(vâ-rô'-nå)

Vicentio
(vê-sen'-shi-ô)

There's plenty of choice here to ensure your kid won't be a chav. Then again, beware of Venice, Verona and Milan; since Brooklyn Beckham, there's every chance a chav might pick a place name for their kid. What you must always bear in mind is that chavs don't think in the same way that we do. A chav thinks not in straightforward monetary terms, but in terms of how much stuff is worth: "How many cans of Stella will that buy me?" "How many pairs of Reebok Classics can I get for one Stone Island jacket?" "If I get a perm and bleach my hair, will I still have enough left for ten Bensons?"

The other risk you run is that the intellectuals among the chavs – those that read the *Daily Star* – may come across some list of popular kids' names and start using perfectly good and normal names for their own kind, thus sullying them for everyone else. The *Star* did us all a disservice when it published the top boys' and girls' names in the UK on 29 December 2004. Just watch how chavs all over the gaff will pick up on them.

BOYS		GIRLS	
1.	Jack	1.	Ellie
2.	Joshua	2.	Emily
3.	Thomas	3.	Sophie
4.	James	4.	Chloe
5.	Daniel	5.	Jessica
6.	Oliver	6.	Katie
7.	Ben	7.	Lucy
8.	Lewis	8.	Amy
9.	William	9.	Megan
10.	Harry	10.	Olivia
11.	Joseph	11.	Charlotte
12.	Charlie	12.	Hannah
13.	Samuel	13.	Emma
14.	Matthew	14.	Ella
15.	Ethan	15.	Grace
16.	Callum	16.	Mia
17.	Luke	17.	Molly
18.	Benjamin	18.	Lily
19.	Ryan	19.	Lauren
20.	George	20.	Holly

This survey of the 300,000 children born in Britain in 2004 showed that David had dropped out of the top 50 for the first time in over 60 years. See, when Beckham left Man United for Real Madrid it was a case of out of sight, out of mind for the UK's chav population. The *Star*'s own spin was that David fell out of favour because of allegations of affairs by Beckham and Blunkett. *SWAYCI* thinks this is unlikely (why would affairs put a chav off?), but chances are that chavs believed it. Those that could read, that is.

Most of the girls' names in the list used to sound quite classy and timeless. Not any more; now we'll have Megans and Sophies running amok in every council estate in Britain. As for the boys, Jack has now been the name of choice for ten years. Come on parents, use your imagination! In the old days, nobody called their son Jack; the name was used only as a nickname for John. Now they're all called Jack. Jack it in, will you? Leave Jack on his Jack Jones for goodness' sake.

Kids who get lumbered with common names by their parents (come on, not Jack, please), can always try to earn nicknames from playground feats. Dredging up our own schoolyard experiences, *SWAYCI* can offer you by way of example "Bazooka" Joe Reeves (known for chewing), Daz "Milky" Willson (milk monitor), Chris "the Cut" Cummins (always grazing his knees), "Pumpkin" Peter Hurst (dropped a vegetable on the way to harvest festival), "Daft" Mick Jennings (bottom of the class) and "Skid" Mark Johnson (once pooed his pants in music and no one ever lets him forget it).

We're sure you can think of plenty more. We have to stop there; we're still too traumatized by all the abusive nicknames we had to put up with. Some of us are teachers now. We've got to put it all behind us.

Now you've got to the end of this chapter, have a quick look at your local paper's name and shame column. See how many of the top 20 names are in it. Told you so!

Sources
www.babynames.org.uk
http://www.urbandictionary.com/define
  php?term=chav&r=f
www.chavscum.com
http://www.pollwizard.com/2591

FAVOURITE BOYS' NAMES

Name	Last Name	Initials

FAVOURITE BOYS' NAMES

Name	Last Name	Initials

FAVOURITE GIRLS' NAMES

Name	Last Name	Initials
_____		
_____		
_____		
_____		
_____		
_____		
_____		
_____		
_____		
_____		
_____		
_____		
_____		
_____		
_____		
_____		
_____		
_____		
_____		
_____		
_____		
_____		
_____		
_____		

FAVOURITE GIRLS' NAMES

Name	Last Name	Initials

TOP TEN NAMES

BOY

1. _____
2. _____
3. _____
4. _____
5. _____
6. _____
7. _____
8. _____
9. _____
10. _____

GIRL

1. _____
2. _____
3. _____
4. _____
5. _____
6. _____
7. _____
8. _____
9. _____
10. _____

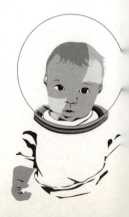